FARRIERY: THE WHOLE HORSE CONCEPT

The enigmas of hoof balance made clear

Farriery: the whole horse concept

The enigmas of hoof balance made clear

David W. Gill

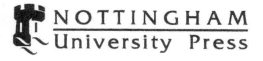
NOTTINGHAM
University Press

Nottingham University Press
Manor Farm, Church Lane, Thrumpton
Nottingham, NG11 0AX, United Kingdom

NOTTINGHAM

First published 2007
Reprinted 2018
© DW Gill

British Library Cataloguing in Publication Data
Farriery: the whole horse concept
I. Gill, David. W.

ISBN   978-1-904761-55-6

Disclaimer

Every reasonable effort has been made to ensure that the material in this book is true, correct, complete and appropriate at the time of writing. Nevertheless the publishers, editors and authors do not accept responsibility for any omission or error, or for any injury, damage, loss or financial consequences arising from the use of the book.

Every effort has been made to obtain permission to reproduce the illustrations in this book. However, if any rights have accidentally been infringed, the publisher would be pleased to hear from the owner to correct the matter.

Typeset by Nottingham University Press, Nottingham
Printed and bound by CPI Group (UK) Ltd, Croydon, CR0 4YY

Contents

6 MEDIOLATERAL HOOF BALANCE   99

7 THE CROOKED HORSE   113

8 FARRIERY IN PRACTICE   127

Background

With an estimated 120 million working horses, donkeys and mules in the world, farriery as a welfare issue is as important today as it has ever been. In the USA alone there are somewhere in the region of 7 million equines, which, when combined with the total number of horses in the English speaking countries of Australia, Canada, New Zealand and the UK amounts to a staggering total of over 11 million animals. With all these animals requiring care and attention, are the farriers who work on those horses truly at ease with their craft and if they are not, why not? Over recent years there has been a rising groundswell of dissatisfaction, fuelled by the free and open access of information available both through the thirst of the popular press and the inexhaustible Internet. Farriers and veterinarians are trained to be expert in their fields but when exposed to the real world quickly realise the textbook horses and scenarios they have been taught to deal with seldom exist: now owners are beginning to realise that too. With this kind of pressure, we all need to stop and reflect.

Farriery is an ancient craft perceived by many as being both quaint and idyllic, immortalised on canvas by famous artists over the centuries; a craft that has remained relatively unchanged for hundreds of years.

Despite the longevity of its practice and the antiquity of its generally accepted principles, the reason farriery has failed to develop at the same pace as other crafts is quite simple. It has been the lack of understanding between those who practice the craft, those who pay for the work and those who sit in judgement.

This has meant it has allowed itself to become stuck in a time warp of cyclical impasse with recurrent variations to its methodology changing only because neither farriers, owners nor veterinarians have ever been truly at ease with the techniques or systems practised. I believe that had there been a different relationship between those responsible for our horses, advances would have been continuous, realised through the technical refinements in the practical application of the craft and the unravelling of biomechanics, encouraged through input from relevant scientific fields.

Throughout the history of farriery, there have been many individuals who have made significant contributions to better our knowledge by setting down their thoughts about this fascinating subject. They have done so driven by the knowledge that although the hand skills of the farrier, which are practised daily, would appear to be quite readily judged; the science behind those skills is largely unproven. Although anyone can see when a horse has lost a shoe, or has become lame after shoeing, understanding why and explaining the reasoning involved, is far more difficult.

Why incidences of lameness and shoe loss occur and how best to shoe a horse to minimise those problems, test farriers on a daily basis. Unfortunately, it has become the tendency of far too many people who do not actually shoe horses themselves, to continually set unrealistic targets of achievement. Such targets supported by ignorance and myth leave some work-conscious farriers in a world of constant failure.

They continue to practice their daily industry knowing that even when they achieve a high standard of workmanship, it can still be viewed as being only that, which is expected of them. Although a farrier's efforts may very well be valued while a horse is untroubled, lame horses and lost shoes are inevitable and so are very much a reality of any normal farriery business.

A different perception of farriery has long been overdue. This may only come about if we who share our concerns about farriery adopt a new approach to those haunting questions that continue to stretch and tease this profession. Our way forward should be based upon reflection and research and include exploring some fields of research previously overlooked or discounted. So to start with, we need to redefine exactly that which we understand as natural, and explain that which is well within the parameters of being considered reasonably acceptable.

Farriers are busy practical people, so the science behind farriery needs to be 'up front' and accessible based upon observable facts, with objectivity and purpose forming the criteria of any judgement or conclusion.

While many authors have taken up the challenge to present their truths in their own fashion, few have found success in having their published works read in the tack-room, the forge and the surgery. This book has been written to appeal to all these relevant audiences. I hope you will find it easy to read and understand and above all, that the book is informative and thought provoking. It is essential we bridge the gulf of understanding between, owner, farrier and veterinary surgeon and develop farriery into the modern progressive profession I am convinced it can and should be.

Back of the beating hammer by which the steel is wrought.
Back of the workshops clamour, the seeker may find a thought.
The thought that is ever master of iron and steam and steel, that rises
*   above disaster and tramples it under heel.*

Back of them stands the schemer, the thinker who drives things
*   through.*
Back of the job, the dreamer who's making the dream come true.

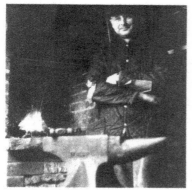

The author: photograph courtesy of Alec Keeper, Nottingham, UK.

The Thinker
By Berton Braley, 1882-1966

Foreword

By Ernie Gray, farrier, speaker and clinician,
Owensville, Ohio, USA

I enjoy a good axiom, and some time ago, I developed this one: "Mistakes are the consequence of effort, experience is the accumulation of mistakes, knowledge is the collection of experience and wisdom is the proper application of knowledge". With the writing of this book, David Gill both exemplifies and demonstrates that he is decidedly capable of the proper application of wisdom that is born of his years of accumulated knowledge and experience.

No stranger to the pen, David Gill has written numerous articles over the years. Anyone who reads his articles is certain to learn from them for they are meticulously researched, craftily written and beautifully and skilfully illustrated. The same can be said of this, his latest and to date most ambitious work, *'FARRIERY: the whole horse concept. The enigmas of hoof balance made clear'*.

Some might say, "why do we need yet another book on horseshoeing"? Generally I would agree, however, I believe that in an excerpt from another classic text on farriery, Leslie Emery both reveals and validates the need with this statement, *"Periodically, the basic principles of a profession must come under careful review. Re-examination of the concepts upon which, one's work is founded is the only path to improvement though not necessarily by invalidating the practices of the past; rather, it should expand upon that work, using it as a base. Our goal in writing this book is to provide both a reappraisal and a new perspective, and to eliminate some contradictions and misconceptions regarding the art of horseshoeing."*

My association with David Gill goes back many years and began as a result of our mutual preoccupation with equine asymmetry. In that time, I have grown to respect and admire him for his dedication to and passion for farrier science, as well as for his skilled accomplishments in both writing and illustration. However, it is with regard to his approach to research that David really excels, for he demonstrates a dogged pursuit of truth and relentless attention to detail that must be viewed not just with respect, but also with awe.

The subject of equine asymmetry, particularly with regard to the question of whether its origins are inherent or acquired, is one that is undeniably controversial. However, despite the controversy or, perhaps more because of it, discussions on the topic are common today, whereas just a few years ago the subject was, for the most part, of little interest to anyone. Today, interest in equine asymmetry, both inherent and acquired is quickly gaining in popularity. As is evidenced by the fact that nearly every clinic, seminar or convention relating to farrier science or veterinary science has at least one speaker on hand to discuss the topic of mismatched feet. Still, the subject of innate equine asymmetry has been given little more than a passing mention in serious contemporary farrier writings. Until now that is.

After years of researching the topic of equine asymmetry, David Gill not only has presented the subject in his new book but also discusses it in great detail. The reader will find that the amount of information and the depth of discussion relating to this subject is far greater than appears in any other book currently on the market.

Don't let me mislead you though, *'FARRIERY: the whole horse concept'* is far more than a treatise on the subject of equine asymmetry, it is the whole package, covering the gambit by providing timely and detailed information for everyone associated with horses. David says it best in another excerpt from his book when he says, *"The main directive behind any such book, is that it has to be both easy to read and easy to understand; a book which is not only accessible but also informative; informative enough to bridge the gulf of understanding between owner, farrier and veterinary surgeon".*

For those who have been searching, *'FARRIERY: the whole horse concept'* has solid, sensible answers for those who desire to know more about how the horse does what it does. In this book, David explains not just about the mechanics but how the anatomy, physiology, bio-mechanics, kinematics and conformation of the horse serve to facilitate function and how all of these things work together organically and mechanically to function according to the rules of nature.

To quote from David Weese's *Life and times of W.M. Harvey,* "Nature tends to perfection, even if man does not, and we ought to consult more with our senses and instinct, than the fashion of the century."

In my opinion, a need exists for a book that re-examines the practices of our profession; eliminating contradictions and misconceptions while at the same time providing accurate information that will serve the horse by informing and educating. I strongly believe that the information in this book is essential for anyone associated with horses and will not only inform and educate but may just serve to realistically bridge the gap between owner, trainer, farrier and veterinarian.

I recommend *'FARRIERY: the whole horse concept'* by David Gill to anyone in the horse industry who is serious about understanding how the horse functions and the role the farrier plays in helping the horse to function properly and soundly.

My thanks to David Gill for his steadfast dedication and seemingly boundless energy in bringing this work to the horse-loving public.

Ernie Gray

Preface

By Kerry J. Ridgway, veterinarian, speaker and horseman,
Aiken, South Carolina, USA

David Gill, in this book, has addressed three major issues that have long been in need of discussion. Just as I start many lectures with the statement that "today's knowledge is tomorrow's misinformation," David has aptly pointed out how we must constantly challenge yesterday's truths, while still using the knowledge to build today's concepts.

He has also accomplished two more important, and in my opinion, critical tasks. He has challenged today's farriers to look at the whole horse, so that they may shoe the horse rather than just shoeing the foot.

Additionally he has addressed the absolute necessity of the veterinarian and farrier developing better understanding, communication and the need to function as a team for the good of the horse.

Kerry J. Ridgway, DVM

Born the son of a horseman Dr Kerry Ridgway has had a lifetime's association with the horse, which has led him to experience and explore many disciplines and practices.

Dr Ridgway is well known to the endurance riding fraternity not only as a veterinarian but also as a competitor and it was through his achievements and contributions to the sport that he was elected to the Endurance Riding Hall of Fame.

He was a founding member and officer for the Association for Equine Sports Medicine, which is now a large international association. However, after practicing conventional medicine for over twenty years, Dr Ridgway developed a deep interest in complementary therapies.

As a certified veterinary acupuncturist and chiropractor, Dr Ridgway has sought to provide the best of both worlds combining these practices with accepted conventional medicine. However, his philosophy extends even further by recognising the impact that other integrated factors, such as farriery, can have upon the 'whole horse'; and it is this enlightened approach to modern veterinary medicine that will shape future therapeutic and rehabilitative procedures.

Acknowledgements —————————————————————

In some ways, it would be easier to mention those who have not had a hand in this book because wherever there has been any interest or an offer of help I've tried to make the best use of it.

Notwithstanding, the first person I should mention is Mr Ken Hathaway, for it was he who first suggested the idea and it was his initial encouragement that got the project started.

Having started I found I needed someone to read my work and Jane Ogilvie stepped in and helped out where she could, but the key worker throughout this undertaking has been my trusted friend Dorothy Fairfax. Without her continued nagging and constant support it would never have got finished.

Others have also been involved; Katy Parkes silently provided me with the drive and much needed incentive to complete, reminding me that to give up at any point would have been to fail.

Nevertheless, the project nearly crashed on many occasions. However, when things were at their absolute lowest and my direction almost gone, a white knight in the form of David Shelton rode by, he cut and pasted some 35k words, seamlessly restructuring the chapters to make them more presentable. It was David's belief in my abilities that gave me a fresh intake of breath and provided me with the confidence to finally complete the work

Lyn Hopegood also lent her support and gave freely of her time, reading through all of the manuscript, making suggestions and amendments where she thought they were needed.

Illustrating and supporting the text with photographs has been an absolute nightmare but, fortunately, John Watts came to the rescue and took some outstanding pictures providing an essential contribution.

This list of people who have helped out and supported could seem endless but like any project that takes over one's life it is those who are the closest who shoulder the largest burden. So, my thanks and apologies go out to them, my family…please bear with me when I start all over again!

My thanks also go out to the many who have listened, helped and encouraged; Samuel Beeley, Louise Berrisford, Doug Bradbury, Marie Brentford, Ann Broughton, Gary Burton, Sally Chiarella, Hilary Clayton, Chris Colles, Melvin Cross, Richard Day, Soleil Dolce, Val Donger, Mark Ellis, Leslie Emery, Pam Farquhar, Gene Freeze, Brian Fuller, Ernie Gray, Scott Gregory, Bonnie Urquhart Gruenberg, Susan

Harris, Barry Higham, Pauline Holloway, Denise Hutchins, Mary Jackson, Justine Jenkins, Sarah Keeling, Sue Kempson, Janet Manning, Terry Martin, Donal McNally, Judith Mulholland, Steve Newman, Shona Nock, Andrew Parks, Adeline Pell, Kerry Ridgway, June Smith, Mary Smith, Pat Thacker, Sarah Tomlinson, Meike van Heel, Ron Ware, Ros Webb and Geraint Wyn-Jones…many thanks to you all and apologies to those I've failed to mention… I could never have done it without you.

The author is a practicing farrier and can be found at:

Millfield Smiddy, Mill Lane, Aslockton,
Nottingham, NG13 9AS, England

www.thefarrierbox.co.uk

1: Introduction

'Philosophy is not a theory but an activity'

Ludwig Wittgenstein 1889 - 1951

What does philosophy have to do with farriery? The answer is – everything! Philosophy is a study of realities and general principles, a study of systems and theories, a principle that calmly investigates the very nature of all things: to philosophise is to think and probe and put to the test. Whether you are student, professor, apprentice, craftsman or interested horse lover, you have probably picked up this book because you are looking for answers. The lack of satisfactory explanations to many questions, which arise while dealing with horses, is both puzzling and frustrating. Perhaps it is just that the right questions have not been asked of the right people at the right times.

Horses have always had hooves and for the last two thousand years or so, farriers have been applying shoes to those hooves in order to protect them from damage. How deeply disappointing it is then that this collective build up of experiences and knowledge has continually suffered from a lack of communication and a strong reluctance to share. It is unfortunate also, as if that wasn't enough, that we have an innate tendency to make things fit into our own level of understanding; we hold back, instead of taking our thoughts that step further and expanding our knowledge and awareness, and this is what we must do.

To make new and real advances in farriery there has to be a general change in our philosophic approach towards this time worn industry. We need to look to the past, question our practices and develop new thinking.

THE BIRTH OF A NEW AGE IN FARRIERY

Over thirty years ago, an apprentice usually started out as a Saturday boy, sweeping floors, making tea and cutting off steel. The industry (if one could call it that) was a way of life, an echo of the past, a sort of living museum, with evocative sights, sounds and smells. It was an industry that was larger than life and built upon folklore and myth (Fig. 1-1).

Farriery, at that time was something of an ancient art; a skill handed down through traditional teaching practices. Therefore, understandably, it was considered by many that it was only those who

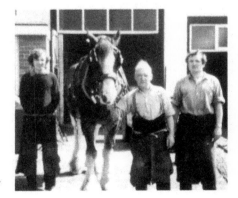

Fig. 1-1: Echoes of the past and the birth of a new age in farriery. The author (left), standing along side the Kimberley Brewery horse, pit blacksmith Alfie Hinsley and master farrier Terry Martin (Photo, courtesy Julie Martin, 1971).

were at least third generation farriers who had the necessary background who knew or understood anything about farriery and in particular hoof balance. So much so, that if any lameness problems occurred, then it was the farrier who was the first person the owner would consult.

Farriers needed to be tough; they worked with steel and fire and flesh. They had to be both strong and confident but despite their self-reliance, they were not blessed with the necessary resources or the background, to discuss veterinary related issues with their sister professionals, the vets. It is unfortunate that this, then and now, has often lead to misunderstandings and at times, frustration on both sides.

Since those times, farriers have tried to establish a new identity for themselves, while some vets have tried desperately to hang on to theirs. The truth is, they are two very different professionals who generally only meet when their roles and relationships are put to a test. Invariably though, it is the owner who has the final say about what they want for their horse. To make rational judgements however, all owners need to be better equipped to know what farriery is and what it is not.

Until fairly recently few books were available to the apprentice farrier. This meant that all skills were passed on from master to apprentice by word of mouth, but only on a need-to-know basis. The main book that was available to farriers at that time ('*The Principles and Practice of Horse-Shoeing* by Charles M. Holmes), looked as if it belonged to an ancient past. In spite of this, it was something not to be questioned and viewed as something akin to the bible.

Back in the early 1970s, there was a steady and continued increase in the role of the horse in leisure pursuits. The equine industry grew and the demand for horse-shoers outstripped availability. Recruitment, training and legislation were then introduced out of necessity to protect horses and save farriery as a craft. Farriery was being reborn and through this rebirth came reflection. In the past, farriers were taught by tradition and tradition by its nature is slow to change. Education was the key, so like good parents, the farriery bodies of the day provided a classroom environment for the new entrants to the trade, albeit for just a few weeks a year. Then after serving a four-year hands-on apprenticeship and passing a stringent trade test, fledgling farriers were let loose upon the world, keen and eager to find and establish a new identity that would embrace the old with the new.

However, not all was well and in the 1980s, farriery entered a new phase. There was a growing concern that many lameness problems were now considered to be caused by those self-same farriers who were once held with such high regard.

Since that period, the thirst for knowledge has continued, and the recognition of what good farriery is and who good farriers are has remained somewhat contraversial. A few helped stimulate both question and thought, with contributions to the British farrier's trade magazine, *Forge* (Fig. 1-2).

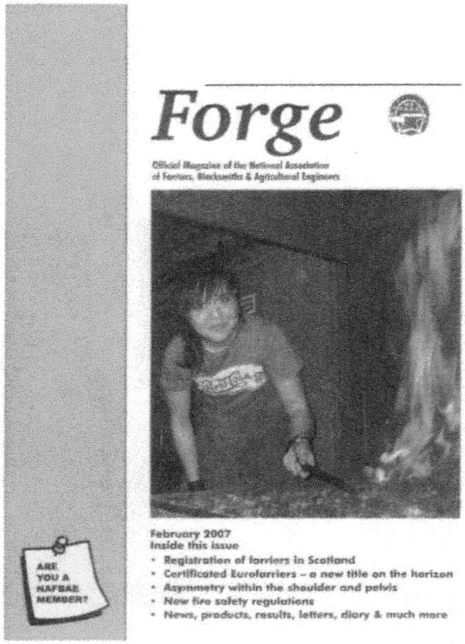

The farriers' trade magazine is the official organ of the National Association of Farriers, Blacksmiths and Agricultural Engineers. Its

Fig. 1-2: *Forge* is a bi-monthly periodical that supports and informs the British farriery industry (image courtesy NAFB&AE, www.nafbae.org).

revered origins go back to 1902, when a small group of regional farriers' associations decided to meet with a view to forming a national body. A conference drawing upon representatives from both England and Wales was held and the result was the creation of 'The National Master Farriers Association'.

The role of the association has always been a welfare role looking after its membership as best it can, sometimes assisted and sometimes hindered by government polices.

Later, the association became the owners of The Farriers Journal Publishing Company and since then this official magazine has continued to be a source of communication between what would otherwise be individuals working in isolation. It has proved to be a valuable asset to the farriery industry as has been the 'Farriers Association', an association that has sought not only to work for the welfare of farriers but also to assist with their continuing education. The 'Association' has always recognised that real education is not simply concerned with collecting information but also with finding the best ways of using that information which has been collected; and so the magazine has become essential reading to all interested in farriery.

METHODOLOGY UNDER THE MICROSCOPE

Hoof balance has been a subject that has intrigued for some time because it is the very essence of farriery. A lack of its understanding can cause the early demise of any equine. Although sincere attempts at defining what is the well-balanced hoof have been made, they have been made in such a way, which suggests that only certain theoretical ideals are acceptable and that anything else is not only to be deplored but also condemned. Inevitably, this obsession with presumed ideals, in turn, means that the farrier is consistently striving to achieve what is often practicably unattainable. To seek a theoretical ideal will not only prove fruitless, because perfection can only exist within the perception of our minds, it can undermine the very integrity of those who seek it.

On closer examination into hoof balance, it would appear that many theoretical ideals upon which farriery is being judged are based upon misguided and unqualified judgements. As with any task, and farriery is no exception, guidelines are essential. However, when these guidelines have been created with little regard to the natural evidence, which can be so readily sought out in the form of morbid specimens and x-rays, they only serve to confuse and degrade the farrier's worth. When dealing with nature there has to be a wider understanding of the limitations of any guides or rules used.

Through the study of horses considered to be abnormal or lame and 'unlevel' many can often be discovered to be quite normal, they just did not fall into the accepted pattern of normality.

Over recent years there has been a huge revival of interest in defining what good practice and what good hoof balance are. From this desire to define the ideal, three main concepts have become the generally accepted benchmarks of what is good farriery and normal conformation; and those three main concepts are:

1.   'A perpendicular line dropped from the centre of rotation of the pedal joint should bisect equally the weight-bearing portion of the foot'.

2.   'All horses which display odd sized hooves are suffering from some misdiagnosed, unresolved flexural deformity'.

3.   'When assessing Mediolateral hoof balance with the use of the T-square, if the foot is not level with the bar then what you are seeing is a hoof which is imbalanced'.

However, not all farriers would agree with those statements and despite what would seem to be an organised pattern of indoctrination, the working farrier is far from being at ease with them, which only serves to confuse farrier, owner and veterinarian. So let us look at those statements again.

1.   'A perpendicular line dropped from the centre of rotation of the pedal joint should bisect equally the weight-bearing portion of the foot' (Fig. 1-3).

This guide is an example of a genuine attempt to provide a means to judge the work of the farrier but unless interpretation is exact, it only leads to both misinterpretation and misrepresentation. Upon close inspection, this rule is difficult to accept and impossible to achieve by hoof trimming alone. In fact, there would appear to be no real unshakeable evidence to support such an exacting statement.

    For many years farriers were taught by traditions influenced by market forces and were shoeing the majority of the animals they worked upon with insufficient length to the heels of the shoes. Quite simply, many farriers who took great pride in their work were shoeing with too short a shoe. The idea being impressed upon them was that if the horses were shod with too much length to their shoe, that would increase the risk of the shoes being lost which cast reflections on their skill as a farrier. Therefore, despite the great majority of farriers priding themselves on the quality of their work, lame horses were on the increase. Looking back this was hardly surprising, as evidence and suggestion drawn from antiquity have indicated that insufficient length to the shoe can increase the risk of navicular disease occurring.

    Navicular disease, now more widely referred to as navicular syndrome, is a crippling lameness caused through damage to the navicular bone and the surrounding tissues and structure. The navicular bone, housed within the hoof, serves to dissipate force and facilitate movement. This dreaded lameness found only in the front hooves is recognised to be associated with poor hoof balance, which can result in either or both, the hyperflexion and the hyperextension of the joint, along with the subsequent damage that can ensue.

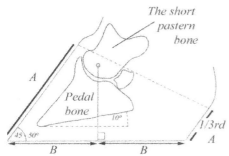

The short pastern bone

Fig. 1-3: A diagram showing the popular conception of the 'ideal balance' for the 'normal foot'.

It is considered that the anterior surface of the hoof wall should run parallel with the wall at the heel, with the heel being 1/3rd the height of the wall at the toe. It is also thought that a perpendicular line dropped from the centre of rotation of the pedal joint should bisect equally the weight-bearing portion of the foot.

Throughout the last few decades, there has been considerable research into the cause and effects of both navicular disease and laminitis, the two most feared causes of lameness, with much of this ongoing investigation being carried out at the Animal Health Trust, Newmarket. The research has been vast and continuous with much of the groundwork being focussed upon hoof balance. It was through this prolonged study that a new concept towards hoof balance was born. In the late 1970s, a new illustration began to appear, firstly in veterinary papers and articles but over the years filtered through onto the pages of the popular press. The origin of this illustration came about through the diligent studies of Chris Colles BvetMed, PhD, HonFWCF, MRCVS; it was an illustration believed to represent both the normal and the desirable hoof. This new concept of what was ideal was the result of the analytical interpretation of a large number of X-rays taken of what were viewed as normal feet. The popularity and acceptance of this abstract idea has grown and developed, though not always however with the knowledge or acknowledgement of what it is based upon or where it came from. Therefore, with its source coming from nature, through the interpretation of someone so highly respected, one could assume its accuracy. However, things being what they are, the original translation of what Chris Colles discovered in the 1970s has frequently become lost. Over time, the illustrations and the suggestion of what others now advocate as both normal and desirable have become less representative of nature and more like stylised impressions, which have evolved and then been fostered by 'Chinese Whispers'. As each artist or author has taken reference from a previous illustration the essence of the analogy has been changed or been made to fit the author's presented plan.

The diagram, which most readers would be familiar with, is the one which appeared in *'Veterinary Notes for Horse Owners'* (Fig. 1-4). In retrospect, it is difficult to appreciate the impact it was to have on the world of farriery. However, when it was published it was probably the first impression of the hoof to show the pedal bone resting at an angle. All previous drawings had always depicted the bone to sit parallel with the ground surface. Interestingly, despite a similar illustration appearing some ten years earlier in *The Veterinary Record*, it was this one, which was to influence the interpretation of many farriers and vets alike when assessing hoof balance.

The accepted notion of anterioposterior balance (AP Balance) starts by assuming that all the past authors had some justification for arriving at their conclusions. However, using some mathematical equations derived from the works of two modern authors, Dr Chris Colles (1993) and Don Birdsall (1990), a more tangible, accessible formula emerges. Based upon their research and understandings, the hoof can be divided into nine sections, with eight of those sections forming an ideal shoe length (Fig. 1-5). Comparing this guide with other documented interpretations of the ideal shoe length it will be found to be a good method to use to emulate exactly what others have, in fact, been promoting.

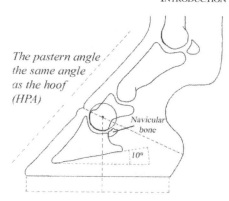

The pastern angle the same angle as the hoof (HPA)

Navicular bone

10°

Fig. 1-4: The accepted example of anterioposterior hoof balance (after the conceptual idea by Chris Colles PhD).

The recognised version of the ideal/normal hoof balance based in accordance with the studies carried out in the 1970s. Hooves not sharing the same proportions have been considered to be deformed by inadequate farriery.

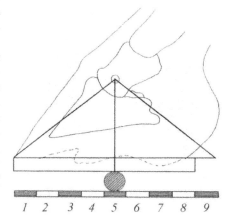

1   2   3   4   5   6   7   8   9

Fig. 1-5: Dividing the hoof into nine equal sections.

Once the hoof has been trimmed, a measurement can be taken, from the bulbs of the heels to the anterior of the toe. From that measurement, we can then divide the hoof into 9 equal sections. The length of eight of those sections can provide us with a guide that will determine an ideal shoe length.

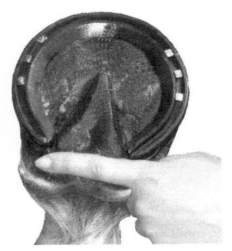

Fig. 1-6: The simple finger guide.

To familiarise yourself with what the shoes look like just after the horse has been shod is essential. Here the finger is used as a guide to judge the distance between the heels of the shoe and the very back of the hoof (the bulbs of the heels).

In farriery, the main consideration is that the hoof is constantly growing. As the hoof grows, the shoe moves forward, ever changing its relationship with the skeletal structure hidden within the hoof. Owners will often notice this growth at the toe of their horse's hooves but the growth seen at the toe is in fact not as critical as the growth which takes place at the heels of the hoof. It is the distance from the back of the foot to the heels of the shoe which must be constantly monitored, because as this distance increases, the support provided by the shoe becomes less. So owners should familiarise themselves with what their horse's hooves look like, just after the farrier has been.

To help us to do that, there is a very simple and handy measuring device available to all, our fingers (Fig. 1-6), with the width of one finger being about 2½cm. When shoes are applied, this is roughly about the distance to leave between the termination of the heels of the shoe and the very back of the hoof. Therefore, when the proverbial two fingers are used to measure that distance, then the horse is desperate for re-shoeing.

2. 'All horses which display odd sized hooves are suffering from some misdiagnosed, unresolved flexural deformity' (Fig. 1-7).

As part of continuous research, one has to constantly consider the aspects of laterality/handedness/asymmetry in the equine and it then becomes clear there is no such thing as the symmetrical horse. Although the idea that symmetry is good is not a bad policy to aim for, the facts are that asymmetry, although something that should not be encouraged, may actually be quite simply a natural phenomenon.

Handedness stirs controversy and debate but although it is increasingly proven to exist, when we read through the index in the back of our veterinary manuals it is not listed. When handedness is discussed the question is raised is it genetic or is it acquired? In one sense the question is irrelevant but an example of inherent asymmetry can be seen in a high proportion of horses as they stand doing what they enjoy best, grazing (Fig. 1-8). This is an act free from manipulation and is a good indicator of which is their dominant side. So, what are the effects of sidedness? Well quite simply it is asymmetry; horses with odd feet are normal, they're just not ideal.

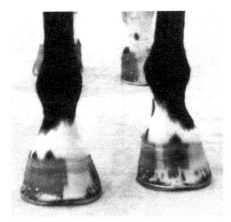

Fig.1-7: A pair of odd sized hooves.

Here the left front foot (to the right of the photo) is considerably smaller and more up-right than the right fore.

These so-called 'mismatched' hooves are frequently described as having an 'unresolved flexural deformity'.

3. 'When assessing Mediolateral hoof balance with the use of the T-square, if the foot is not level with the bar then what you are seeing is a hoof which is imbalanced' (Fig. 1-9).

Mediolateral hoof balance is one aspect of farriery, which is normally limited to one or two paragraphs and with the exception of one author (Gene Freeze, 'Are your horse's feet correctly balanced') - its proper understanding has never developed since William Russell first published his book in 1879.

Practical Scientific Horseshoeing (Russell's book) was rediscovered by Reuel Darling and reprinted in 1988. Russell promoted a symmetry theory stating that the equines legs should be set 'plumb under the body' and that for the joints to work properly the hoof should be trimmed according to a device, which he was marketing, and that was his 'scientific leg and foot tester'. Despite his claims one wonders if in fact he ever actually used the device because he suggested that a different reading would be noted depending upon whether the pastern 'turned in' or 'turned out', when it is highly unlikely that it would make any discernible difference to note. The device when used on the forelimbs, was to be laid down the back of the tendons, with its lower end placed across the heels, that section would then determine if the foot was level or not. The idea that the hoof had to be trimmed according to its relationship with the cannon bone was born. As the reprint began to circulate within the farriery community the idea began to catch on and it was then not long before some of the UK's leading farriers adopted the T-square as their 'definitive guide' to Mediolateral hoof balance. However, the logic behind it is questionable and open to reasoned debate. Therefore, it is hoped, this book should be able to redress some of that which has gone before and help the reader to make more accurate judgements about hoof balance.

The T-square is a tool, which when placed along the back of the cannon bone is used to guide the farrier's assessment of how to trim the hoof. The theory behind its usage is that it acts as a visual aid to check that the ground surface of the foot is at right angles to the cannon or the long axis of the limb. If only hoof balance could be as simple as that, but then the reasoning behind its usage is as naively simple!

Supporters of the T-square theory have made in the past the analogy of likening the hoof and limb to the legs on a table. Suggesting that if the horse were a table, with a leg at each corner and we were to saw each leg off square, then the table would rest level with the floor. The problem with that analogy is that the limb is a 'sophisticated lever or cam system' (Wilson *et al.*, 2003) and that the hoof capsule itself is plastic in its nature. An example of how fallible the theory is can be found in the video 'In Balance', which was issued to all registered British farriers. In the video, a farrier is depicted trimming a hoof with a 'resident Mediolateral imbalance' using a T-square. Later that same farrier informs us that after ten or fifteen minutes the hoof may come 'back over balance' and so no longer remain as initially trimmed. The fact is that the hoof during weight bearing can and does change shape. So, should the T-square be used to judge hoof balance? Well only if our horses are as wooden and lifeless as tables.

When assessing hoof balance we need to have guides, however when those guides become rules there is a danger that in turn these rules will become procrustean in their nature. The T-square has been used as an over simplification and misinterpretation of the evidence. The limb is complex and complex machines are structured by simple components. However to think of the interphalangeal joints as being like door hinges, as some authors have suggested, does not do the mechanism justice. The joints act as cams, with the distal surfaces that form these joints acting as a profile to transmit motion, with the proximal ends forming reciprocating followers. In effect, what this means is that the relationship between the axis of each bone is under

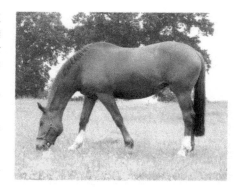

Fig. 1-8: The grazing stance

This is what horses like doing most of all, grazing.

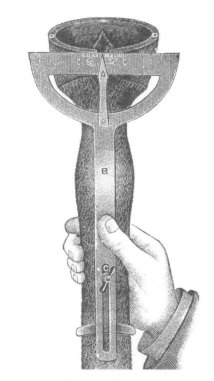

Fig. 1-9: A diagram showing the popular symmetry theory for defining the ideal/normal mediolateral hoof balance (taken from Russell, 1903).

'When assessing mediolateral hoof balance with the use of the T-square, if the foot is not level with the bar then what you are seeing is a hoof which is imbalanced'.

constant change whilst any movement occurs. So how should we judge Mediolateral balance? It is hoped that as the reader becomes more aware and the theories become more transparent then a more reliable plan will become obvious.

FUNDAMENTALS OF FARRIERY

Farriery is a hard, physically demanding, dangerous and sometimes thankless job. Owners are not always aware of this aspect of farriery nor do they understand what they could do to appreciate farriers and farriery more fully than they already do. Many owners already feel that they do their best, tie the horses up ready for the farrier, make him, or her, cups of tea and pay what the farrier asks - what more can they do? Well it is a good start and providing manageable horses in clean safe environments does make the role of the farrier more bearable but it still does not make it easy work. Hard work and farriery are synonymous with one another and although that may never change, when owners realise that farriers shoe because they are dedicated to their craft and they themselves become more knowledgeable about the tasks farriers perform, then the farriery industry itself will improve.

It is essential therefore that all owners acquire an obligation to equip themselves with enough practical know-how to be able to identify good farriery and recognise when their horse's hooves are in need of attention. Likewise good farriers and vets should take it upon themselves to help provide the owners with the means to do so.

Communication is the key to better relations and mutual understanding, so this book will begin by establishing a common language. Unfortunately, farriers, owners and vets do not always appear to speak the same language so it is important to spend a chapter reviewing some essential anatomy and looking at comparative anatomy also. After which a detailed look at the act of farriery will also prove to be essential.

Once the basics are established, this book should guide the reader through the various methodologies employed in farriery today and we shall continue to discuss further those aspects of hoof balance previously outlined within this chapter.

COMMON CONUNDRUMS

The advocates of Natural Balance and Barefoot Trimming techniques have become the latest critiques of modern farriery. Their origins can be traced back to the wild horse studies carried out in the arid regions of the American west by the professional horseman and farrier Jim Miller and the internationally respected veterinarian the late Nyles Van Hoosen. Together they noted and defined naturally shaped hooves; 'shaped by nature in the most natural climate' and so it was that the hooves of the wild mustang horses they studied were to become their blueprint for optimal form and function.

The free exchange of shared knowledge obtained from their professions coupled with their extended relationship with farrier Leslie Emery culminated in the publication of *Horseshoeing Theory and Hoof Care*, (1977). This classic thought-provoking book came as a breath of fresh air challenging many to question old long-established practices. However, its legacy is possibly not as they intended. Certainly they cast their stone and the ripples created a new tide of radical thinking but like so many ideas and theories there are always those who, having had their eureka moments, plagiarised those famed inspired ideas and chose to look no further. There were those also who, rather than embrace the ethos behind the reflective practices of Emery, Miller and Van Hoosen, chose simply to take details of their work and use their ideas as add-ons to their own existing practices. There is no doubt however that this book was to have a profound effect upon the world of modern farriery. It was their organised questioning, designed to make farriers look more closely at nature, that provoked the inception of two different but connecting hoof care strategies, 'Natural Balance' shoeing and 'Barefoot' trimming.

'Breakover' is an important feature of the natural balance systems of shoeing and trimming, yet it is an aspect which is glossed over very easily. It is as if all farriers, vets and owners are considered to know exactly what the phrase means and know exactly what process it describes. However, judging by the total lack of detailed information to be found upon this subject, it is clear that really they are all not too sure about what the functions are that actually take place (Fig. 1-10). Therefore, this too is a subject which requires a review of information and a more detailed explanation if the reader is to become better informed.

'Natural Balance' shoeing (Fig. 1-11) involves placing the shoe much further back under the hoof than conventional shoeing in order to 'ease' breakover. Breakover being the phase occurring in the moments between the time when the hoof is flat on the ground and when the hoof is projected through the air in forward progression. It defines the time when the heels lift off the ground and the toe of the hoof is pushed into the ground surface. The theory behind that line of thought is that by 'easing' the breakover through radically reducing toe length, strain on tendons and ligaments should be reduced. However, the questions of what is normal, what is tolerable and what is essential, are questions that all need to be given equal amounts of in-depth study. To focus on only one aspect of balance or motion in isolation, as many seem to do, is to lose sight of progression and balance as a whole.

Barefoot advocates also focus upon breakover, often in an embellished anecdotal, unscientific way. Their attention is mainly confined to reproducing what they say is a distinct wear pattern, which happens to be a product of the equines going without shoes. Followers of barefoot practices have reported that in certain environmental conditions many horses develop a raised zone around the edge of the hoof's sole, which they describe as a sole callus (Figs. 1-12). Gene

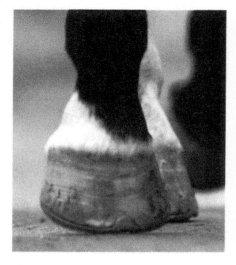

Fig. 1-10: Breakover (photo J. Watts)

'Breakover' is the phrase given to the action, which takes place as the toe of the hoof or shoe becomes a pivotal surface, as the body of the horse passes over the foot during progression. Therefore, it is normal for wear to occur at the lateral aspect of the toe quarter.

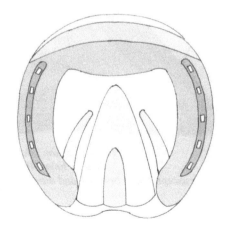

Fig. 1-11: 'Natural Balance' shoeing (after Gene Ovnicek, 1997).

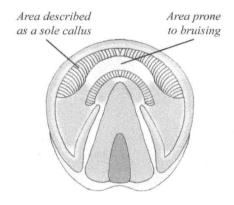

Area described
as a sole callus

Area prone
to bruising

Figs. 1-12: Sole callus
(After Gene Ovnicek, 1997).

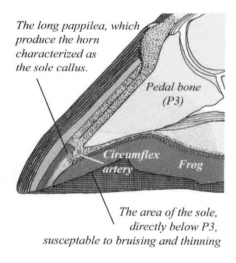

The long pappilea, which
produce the horn
characterized as
the sole callus.

Pedal bone
(P3)

Circumflex
artery

Frog

The area of the sole,
directly below P3,
susceptable to bruising and thinning

Ovnicek, a leading figure within the barefoot and natural balance movement, describes this apparent occurrence as being due to '*a specialised area of sole which grows around the front edge of the coffin bone*'. Interestingly, immediately behind this raised zone is another distinct area, an area, which dependent upon both hoof and environmental conditions is susceptible to bruising. However both seemingly different observations may be caused by the same mechanical actions as both are due to the fact that the hoof is constructed of dermal tissue and is, in simple terms, just a thick piece of skin! The wall of the hoof can and does change shape and so too can the sole of the hoof but to understand the intricacies and the simplicities of the actions that effect these changes we need to look more at the mechanics involved.

One subject, which is essential to all concerned with farriery, is lameness after shoeing. This is a very daunting prospect for the farrier though understandably it is generally more distressing for both the horse and owner. Every time a horse is shod, or trimmed, there is always a risk of it going unsound afterwards, so having a better understanding of what it is like to apply metal to living tissue would prepare the owner for what inevitably will happen at some time. Barefoot practitioners would suggest that all shoeing is damaging but despite this stance they also acknowledge that hoof trimming alone can and does at times cause problems, in fact some groups even openly state that hoof soreness and abscesses are common in the transition from shod hoof to barefoot.

Once upon a time farriery was a clear-cut issue but today it would seem a riddle. Shoeing techniques evolve as individual farriers adapt and refine their skills through experience. They are led by their own passion and the market forces surrounding their localised world. Growing unrest leads to revolution and when revolution takes hold, differing factions and leaders emerge. Conventional farriery, natural balance shoeing and barefoot advocates argue their points. Each have their virtues but we must continually recognise that one compartmental plan will not suit all.

Whether applying shoes, or trimming hooves to go barefoot, the intricacies of the mechanics and nature of hoof and limb need to be constantly considered by all. It's unfortunate, however, that sometimes vets, who should know better, as well as owners, would seem to have little understanding of what can go wrong and why; yet it all comes down to the same thing. The farrier deals with life and flesh, and nature is always there ready to trip you up and kick you when you least expect it.

Abscesses occur from time to time and this is the most common cause of lameness that the farrier is likely to deal with (Figs. 1-13). Despite the frequency of this, there would seem little explanation given of what they are, how they occur and what the treatment is and more importantly, whom the owner should call in.

Lameness from an abscess can be very severe, so severe that sometimes when the owner first notices the problem a fracture is often mistakenly suspected. There is usually heat in the foot, increased pulse and swelling to the lower leg.

More often than not, the farrier is the first to find and expose the abscess. Some vets actually recommend that the farrier is initially called in if an abscess is suspected. This is because farriers tend to be more proficient in finding an abscess and also have the skills needed to open and drain the abscess without damaging healthy tissue. So how do they occur? Well puncture wounds are thought to be the most common injuries; these occur when sharp objects such as old nails, flint or thorns penetrate the sole of the hoof and carry with them infectious agents such as bacteria. The good thing about abscesses is that despite the lameness being acute, once the abscess has been drained recovery can be effective within days. However, even if the farrier is the person who drains the abscess veterinary advice should always be sought.

Prevention of abscesses would seem to be an impossible task but regular attention and monitoring by a professional farrier would seem to be the best course of action. Leaving shoes on for too long without being repositioned by the farrier will cause damage and that could lead to abscessing, so too will leaving unshod hooves without their hooves being rebalanced. In fact, although the idea behind all equines going barefoot is sold as both a prevention and cure for all lameness, interestingly abscesses due to hoof imbalances are reportedly the main reason behind the premature deaths of wild mustangs, which proves nature itself is not as benign as we may think it is.

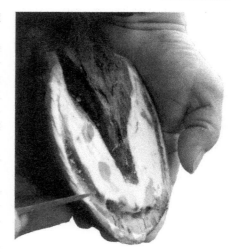

Figs. 1-13: Foot abscesses are a common source of lameness.

One of the most frequent sites is the laminal area commonly known as the white line (as pictured above and below) but puncture wounds are also another regular cause.

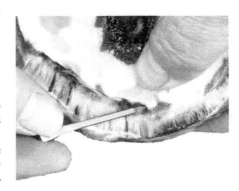

A NEW PHILOSOPHY

It is known that for over two thousand years metal shoes have been applied to horses' hooves. Applying shoes to hooves is not simply a fashion; it is here to stay.

The types of horses in use today, the type of work they do, and the environment in which they live, along with the management they receive, all affect whether they are better with, or indeed are healthier without shoes.

Farriery is often projected as a facility needed to correct imperfect hooves and limbs but before using farriery as a means to right something which is considered to be wrong, the question needs to be asked, are modifications to the hooves the only management those horses require?

Inadequate shoeing and indifferent farriers are frequently cited as being responsible for lameness but what is inadequate shoeing and who are indifferent farriers and who is responsible for their making?

Owners need to recognise their role in farriery is an active one; becoming more than an interested horse lover is essential to equine management and integral to the horse's welfare. All involved in farriery need to be aware that 'corrective' farriery is not about 'quick fixes' and that instant changes do not mean permanent benefits. Farriery is a team effort and hooves need to be managed. Farriery does not begin and end with attaching shoes to horses' feet, having a clear appreciation of what farriery can do is something that needs to be established. A wealth of knowledge, gained through experience and tempered with understanding, will form the basis to any new and successful approach adopted by today's modern freethinking farriers and owners. With us all working together mistakes will then become a thing of the past and the sound horse a product of today.

BIBLIOGRAPHY

'If you take ideas from one source it's called plagiarism. When you take ideas from five its called research'

Birdsall, D., 'Hoof Balance: Definition and measurement with respect of hoof balance', *Forge* (The Farriers' Journal Publishing Co. Ltd February 1990, p.7, 9, 12)

Colles, C. M., Jeffcott, L. B., 'Laminitis in the horse', *The Veterinary Record* (March 1977)

Colles, C., 'Hoof Anatomy and Function', *Horsetalk* (Winter 1993, p.6-9)

Curtis, S. J., Johnson, R. F., 'Foot balance: the WCF view', *Forge* (The Farriers' Journal Publishing Co. Ltd October 1999)

Gill, D. W., 'Hoof Balance: A working Farrier's Interpretation', *1st UK Farriery Convention Handbook* (Equine Veterinary Journal Ltd, 2001, p.59-60)

Hartgrove, T., 'Lameness in Wild Horses and Mustangs; Beyond Natural Balance' (17th Annual Bluegrass Laminitis Symposium 2004 *Journal of Equine Veterinary Science, Volume 24, Issue 7, July 2004, p. 278-284)*

Hayes, M. H., Rossdale, P. H., *Veterinary Notes for Horse Owners* (Stanley Paul & Co. Ltd 1988, p.292-304)

Holmes, C. M., *The Principles and Practice of Horse-Shoeing* (The Farriers' Journal Publishing Co. Ltd 1949)

'History of the Association', *National Association Farriers, Blacksmiths & Agricultural Engineers* (Handout Publication)

'In Balance: Hoof Trimming for Competitiveness and Work', *A Farriers Guide to the Basics of Good Hoof Trimming* (Farriers Registration Council, 1999)

Ovnicek, G., *New Hope for Soundness* (Equine Digit Support System, Inc. 1997)

Russell, W., *Practical Scientific Horseshoeing* (Loose Change Publications, 1987)

Ryan, T., 'Shaping up for a sounder footing', *Horse & Hound* (12th June 1997, p.66-67)

Simons, M. A. P., 'The future of farriery', *The Veterinary Record* (January 1976, p.72-73)

Strasser, H., Hoof Abscesses. http://www.thehorseshoof.com/abscesses.html (Access March, 2007)

Williams, G. and Deacon, M., *No Foot, No Horse* (Kenilworth Press Ltd, 1999)

Wilson, A. M., Watson, J. C., Lichtwark, G. A., 'A catapult action for rapid limb protraction', *Nature* (January 2003, p.35-36)

Wright, I. M., Douglas, J., 'Papers and Articles', *The Veterinary Record* (July 1993, p.109-114)

2: Anatomy explained

BUILDING A COMMON LANGUAGE

At the beginning of any inquiry, it is essential to establish a common understanding or language. Often communication between owner, farrier and vet is hindered simply because of the lack of any real knowledge shared between all three parties. This chapter will therefore form the groundwork for establishing the basics of an essential common awareness needed for all parties to communicate. It is not intended that this chapter or book should replace the need to source reference from other material but rather it should encourage you, the reader, to seek out other, more detailed texts. This section is essentially here to help clarify certain points in order to make the other chapters within this book easier to understand.

What fundamentally divides farriers and their clients is that neither is fully aware of each other's perceptions and interpretations. The owner often knows very little about even the basic of tasks that the farrier has to perform and usually has no concept at all of what it is like to go from one struggling horse to another. The farrier on the other hand sometimes has very little knowledge of how the owner genuinely views his role. The farrier/vet divide likewise usually exists for similar reasons. Often, the farrier feels that the vet views him only as a technician, expected to carry out certain instructions, frequently without any real consultation. However, the divide that exists between the three parties, whatever it may be, when recognised can begin to dissolve, as we all should have the shared aim of the welfare of the horse at heart. It is possible that we can all be interested experts who all communicate in a shared common language.

THE LINKS BETWEEN MAN AND HORSE

The horse is a single hoofed quadruped, which effectively stands upon its middle finger (Fig. 2-1). The horse, as we know it, has been around for thousands upon thousands of years. The links in terms of the relationship of man and horse has been lost within the mist of time. However, references can be found to the existence of the horse in Chinese tradition dating as far back as 2348 BC. Regarding the origins of the horse today, available information suggests that reliable scientific research has been unable to establish the precise common ancestral link between horses, donkeys and zebras. Despite this,

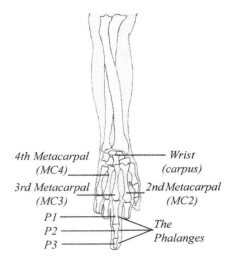

4th Metacarpal (MC4) — Wrist (carpus)

3rd Metacarpal (MC3) — 2nd Metacarpal (MC2)

P1, P2, P3 — The Phalanges

Fig. 2-1: The human hand

The horse effectively stands upon its middle finger, with the bones of the equines lower limb being a homologue of the human hand. The bones of the human hand and the corresponding bones of the horse's lower limb comprise of the second, third and fourth metacarpals, and the first, second and third phalanges.

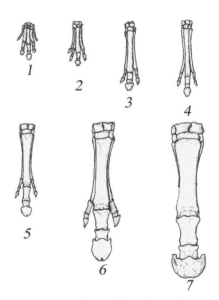

Fig. 2-2: The illustrations 1-7 depict the evolutionary transition from the horse's ancestral five-toed predecessor to the modern single toed horse of today.

1. Phenaeedus
2. Protorohippus
3. Mesohippus
4. Miohippus
5. Protohippus
6. Hipparion
7. Horse

collectively, these similar animals are considered to form the equidae group of mammals. The equidae are a group of mammals linked because they all share the same characteristic feature and it is this single feature, which defines this family from all other ungulates. Ungulates are the families of all hooved animals such as sheep, goat, pig, cattle and horse. Uniquely the feature that separates the equidae from all the other hooved mammals is the fact that it is only the third digit which comes into contact with the ground forming a single functioning hoof. While the remainders of the second and fourth digits still survive from a prehistoric evolutionary era, these have become greatly reduced in both size and function (Fig. 2-2). All that now remains of those lost digits are the **second** and **fourth metacarpal** bones, of which, the **proximal** ends (or the upper ends) serve to provide an area of articulation with the bones of the knee.

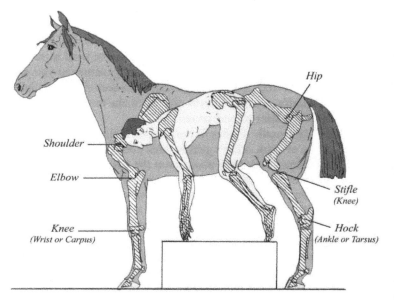

Fig. 2-3: Comparative anatomy (After Duhousset, 1896,who based his illustration upon the idea suggested by Garsant in his book the *New Complete Farrier*, 1769).

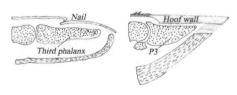

Fig. 2-4: The human fingernail and the horse's hoof both serve to shield and protect the third of the phalangeal bones, which form the extremity of the human and equine digit.

To trace the origins of the horse back to some decisive dawning would be an impossible task. However, it is important for us all to know and understand that there are associations between the species and that the links between all animals exist through their common ancestry. This pool of common ancestry connects all mammals, both equines and humans alike. Indeed, if we were to look back millions of years, it is probable that we all evolved from some fish-like creatures and it is because of these primordial genetic associations that certain likenesses can be found (Fig. 2-3). In fact, when describing the horn of the hoof it is quite common, by a wide variety of people, to refer to it as being like our fingernail and they have a very good reason for making that analogy, because it is.

TERMINOLOGY OR ANATOMICAL NOMENCLATURE

The terminologies within the farriery and veterinary worlds are, just as is the English language, in a constant state of flux, ever changing. The academic authorities and nomenclature committees suggest that this occurs in order to identify and isolate a precise phrase given to an exact meaning. However, often these phrases rather than help identify, create obstacles and obstruct both learning and understanding. Therefore, throughout this chapter it is hoped that you will be encouraged to expand your vocabulary so that we can all share our knowledge without stumbling over words or phrases, which at present may seem very foreign.

Most of you will be familiar with certain phrases, which identify the various aspects of the body. Some of those phrases and aspects will need no identification or explanation but others will, so for the purpose of this text, only certain features will be examined and only those considered pertinent will be examined in any detail.

THE MEDIOLATERAL VIEW EXPLAINED

When viewing the horse, looking at it from the front most lay people will use the term 'head on'. However, when that view is used to describe the angle at which an x-ray beam may be focussed upon a film plate, then it is called a *craniocaudal* view, *cranial* appertaining to the head and *caudal* appertaining to the tail. Although this phrase is frequently used to describe this view, the term *anterioposterior* is also used (Fig. 2-5); again, this comes from the way in which the point of entry of an x-ray beam will be focussed *anteriorly* upon a patient and exit *posteriorly* on to a film plate. *Anterior* is a phrase given to something, which is situated or directed towards the front of an object, and is directly opposite to the *posterior*, *postero* being a word element taken from the Latin meaning back. Where the view is the opposite, viewing an object from the back towards its front, then that view may be described as a *posteroanterior* view (Fig. 2-6). In quadrupeds, animals that have four feet, the term anterior is generally limited to parts of the head but is often used to mean *cranially*, or towards the front. When the horse is standing squarely and the observer is assessing either hoof or limb balance from an anterioposterior plane, then the terms *medial* or *lateral* are used. The phrase medial appertains to an aspect close to the centre, or midline, of the animal and lateral denoting an aspect further from the midline, toward its outer side. Therefore, when assessing hoof or limb balance in that plane it is often referred to as a *mediolateral* balance assessment.

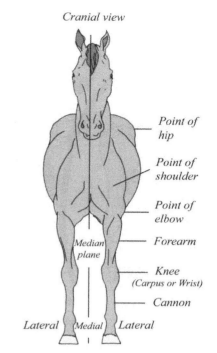

Cranial view

Point of hip

Point of shoulder

Point of elbow

Forearm

Knee (Carpus or Wrist)

Cannon

Median plane

Lateral Medial Lateral

Fig. 2-5: Anterioposterior view, (after Duhousset, 1896).

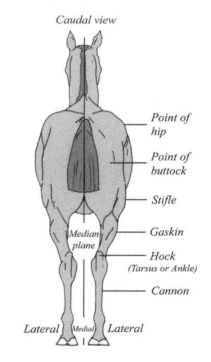

Caudal view

Point of hip

Point of buttock

Stifle

Gaskin

Hock (Tarsus or Ankle)

Cannon

Median plane

Lateral Medial Lateral

Fig. 2-6: Posteroanterior view, (after Duhousset, 1896).

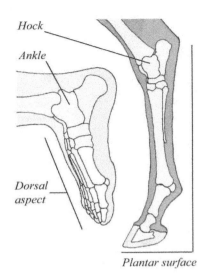

Fig. 2-8: Comparisons can be made between the human foot and the horse's hind limb (after Axe, 1905)

THE ANTERIOPOSTERIOR VIEW EXPLAINED

When viewing the horse from the side, this view is frequently described as a lateral view (Fig. 2-7). Lateral is a phrase denoting a presence located away from the midline, or the *median plane* of a body or structure, so lateral refers to an object being to one side of any medial plane. Lateral views are used to assess equine hoof balance in an anterioposterior plane. This type of assessment is also frequently described as *dorsopalmar* balance, *dorso*, being derived from the Latin word element meaning back or *dorsal*. The term dorsopalmar is used in veterinary practice to describe the passage of an x-ray beam from the dorsal aspect of the forelimb through to its *palmar* aspect. In the horse, the front of the limb is referred to as the dorsal aspect and the back of the limb is referred to as the palmar aspect of the limb. However, in the case of a hind limb this view is known as a *dorsoplantar* view, although this method of identification is limited to the limbs below the knee and hock. Here an appreciation of comparative anatomy (Fig. 2-3) helps to understand the meanings of these phrases and helps put equine anatomy on grounds that are more familiar. The segment of the limb, which is referred to as the equine's knee, or *carpus*, is in dogs, cats and humans always known as the *wrist*. The back of our hands in medical terms is referred to as the dorsal aspect: and our palms? Well they help us to remember that the back of the equine's forelimb, from the carpus or wrist down is known as the palmar aspect. Likewise, just as the soles of our feet are medically known as the *plantar* surfaces, the equine's hindlimb from the *hock* down, which can be compared to our *ankle*, is known as the plantar aspect (Fig. 2-8).

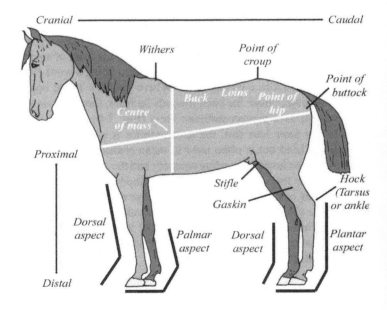

Fig. 2-7: A lateral view of the horse, (after Duhousset, 1896).

So when taking all this background information on board, when we consider hoof balance viewing the hoof from a lateral plane, this type of assessment will be referred to, in this text, as *anterioposterior* hoof balance. However, when referring to the front of the hoof and limb this may be described as either anterior or dorsal. When discussing the back of the limb this may be referred to as the posterior, the palmar or the plantar aspects.

THE EXTERIOR OF THE HORSE

Describing the equine's exterior, moving around the body starting from the head and descending down the neck along the top-line of the animal there is to be found the point known as the *withers* (Fig. 2-9). This is the highest point of the thoracic spine and is formed by the third to fifth thoracic vertebrae, where the dorsal margins of the *scapula* (shoulder blade) lie just below the skin. Continuing along the top-line of the animal past the loins, there is a prominence known as the *croup* (Fig. 2-10). This feature is the region which covers the two sides of the pelvic bone called the *ilium*; these two eminences are identified and named as the *tuber sacrale*.

Following the gluteal mass, forming the rump which covers the pelvic region, descending past the dock of the tail, there is another prominent feature known as the *point of buttock*, here the flesh covers that part of the pelvis known as the *seat bone* or *tuber ischium*. From this point, moving down the limb distally the *point of hock* will be found (Fig. 2-11); this feature forms part of the tarsus or ankle joint. Below this joint, the back of the hind limb is referred to as the plantar aspect and all the joints (of which there are three in number) are considered to belong to the lower or *distal* aspect of the limb. The first of those distal joints, which make up the limb, is the *fetlock,* which is quite noticeable, while the two others that articulate the phalanges are almost indistinguishable. The *pastern* joint having little form as it takes in only a small range of motion and the *pedal* joint, or *coffin* joint, also known as the distal *interphalangeal* joint, being partially hidden by the *hoof capsule*. The underside of those hooves belonging to the hind limbs may be referred to as the plantar surface or *solear surface* of the foot.

Moving along to the anterior of the hoof and continuing *proximally* up the limb, this aspect below the hock is known as the dorsal surface of the limb. The term *proximal* is a phrase used here to describe a site or point closest to the centre of the body, whereas a site or point furthest away may be described as being distal from any such reference point. Above the hock is the aspect of the limb known as the *gaskin* or second thigh, (the equivalent of the human calf). Stashak (1976) refers to it as being the crus, or true leg. The joint above the gaskin and hock located in the upper or proximal half of the hind limb is the equivalent of our knee and is known as the *stifle*, which features the *patella*.

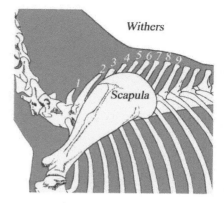

Fig. 2-9: The withers

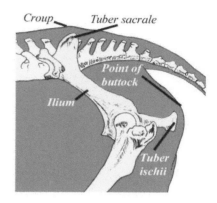

Fig. 2-10: The croup

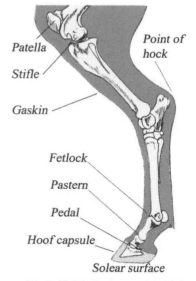

Fig. 2-11: The hock and distal limb

19

THE CENTRE OF MASS

Continuing forward under the main body or trunk of the animal, travelling cranially towards the forelimbs, there is a location within the body of the animal, which is not a simple theoretical notion but is an axis point, which is both ill defined and dynamic. It's called the *centre of mass* or *centre of gravity* (Fig. 2-12) and it plays a huge part in the balance and equilibrium of any equine and as such, its importance and approximate location should always be considered. It has been suggested that it is located somewhere at a point situated between the point of the shoulder and the point of the buttock. Some consider its location to be variable but if an imaginary line is strung between those two points and it is then (in the standing horse) bisected by a line dropped from the animal's withers, then that will approximate its location. Its role in farriery has not always been fully considered and yet its continuous influence upon the equine limb and hoof is always profound. Although its effects have failed to be totally recognised, the consequence of its involvement in equine conformation has perplexed both farriers and veterinary surgeons for generations.

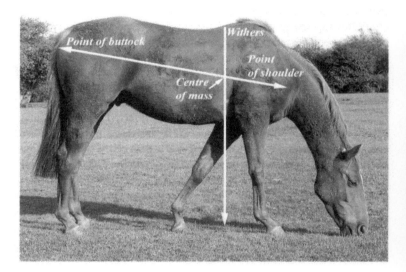

Fig. 2-12: The centre of mass is located at some point behind the withers.

The centre of gravity is thought to have first been described by the mathematician and anatomist Alphonso Borelli, in his book published in 1681. In fact, it is probably because of his work, when in describing the gaits of the horse, that movement is said to first begin with the placement of a hind limb. Borelli suggested that walk began with the lifting and positioning of a hind foot, his reasons for describing this theory was that if a fore foot were lifted, that would disturb the animal's centre of gravity and therefore that action would be too destabilising.

Researchers have acknowledged the existence of the centre of gravity for quite sometime and a number of those researchers have gone to great lengths to establish its location. Goubaux and Barrier, French veterinary surgeons were said to have carried out extensive research, the results of which were included into their book 'The Exterior of the Horse' (1882). The type of research they adopted (and others have since replicated), has included a live horse standing on scales and suspending an embalmed body from a cable until it balanced. However, the location of the centre of mass, which they set out to establish, varies within each individual horse and that too it is thought, will also change with every given moment as stance and movement influences its location. For example, it is suggested that during the act of grazing, the placement of the horse's hooves and the movement of the head and neck will cause the centre of mass to move and that in turn will affect the force on the hooves and limbs. When the head is lowered, the centre of mass moves forward, when it is lifted, the centre of mass moves backwards. So whether the centre of mass moves or not, the force upon the limbs is bound to be affected. This will occur because during the act of grazing, as Stewart Hastie in his book suggests, one forelimb is flexed (the hoof placed in advance of the body), so becoming 'shorter', while the other forelimb is extended and takes support (Fig. 2-13). This action allows the trunk and the base of the neck to sink nearer the ground to facilitate the act of grazing. The products of those combined actions then influences hoof shape because the limb that is extended (that is the limb of which the distal joints are fully extended) is placed either beneath or behind the body's centre of mass. Force then compresses the horn of the hoof dorsally (at the toe), while the hoof belonging to the limb stretched out in front, the limb that is the more flexed, is compressed palmarly (at the heels).

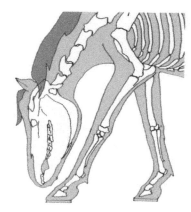

Fig. 2-13: During the act of grazing the equines centre of mass moves forward.

As the limb, which is placed in advance of the body (protracted) is stretched out, the distal limb becomes flexed, whereas the other leg, which is placed under the body (retracted) has its distal limb placed in an extended position.

This action causes force to be applied the heels of the protracted hoof and the toe of the retracted hoof.

THE EXTERIOR OF THE HORSE CONTINUED

Continuing with the identity of the exterior parts of the body, (Fig. 2-14) moving forwards under the equine's belly can be found a feature of the forelimb; the *elbow*. The joint situated below the elbow is the *knee* and from that point, the back of the knee and the posterior surface below is known as its palmar aspect. The posterior aspect of the distal limb below the knee is termed the palmar surface and this continues down past the fetlock, the pastern and the pedal joint and includes the ground, or solear surface of the hoof. The anterior or front of the hoof and distal limb is also known as its dorsal aspect and this term extends proximally until the dorsal aspect, or front of the knee is reached. The portion of the limb above the knee is called the *forearm* and this region lies between the knee and the elbow. Finally, we arrive at the point of the *shoulder*.

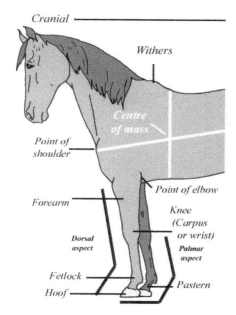

Fig. 2-14: The exterior of the horse continued, (after Duhousset, 1896).

THE SKELETAL FRAMEWORK OF THE HORSE

To get a better perception of how these exterior features relate to the equine's form and function it would be useful to have x-ray vision, which unfortunately none of us possess. However, fortunately the bones of any animal are a lasting indicator and a tangible reminder that the skeleton forms a strong internal framework around which the soft body hangs (Fig 2-15).

The skeleton supports the body, anchors the muscles and protects the vital organs. The shape and form of bones are enduring elements, which can reveal secrets about any animal's way of life and style of moving, so much so that palaeontologists, archaeologists and anthropologists use the bones to build up a picture of the principles of existence of creatures and people long gone. A closer look at those bones that make up the equine limbs allows us to get a better perception of how farriery relates to that structure.

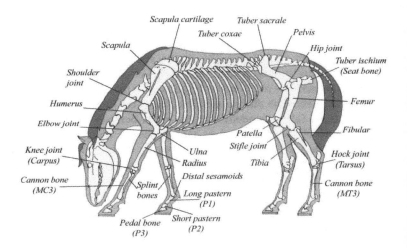

Fig. 2-15: The skeletal framework of the horse (after Elliott, *The New Dogsteps*, 1983).

BONE

Bones are complex living structures, which both support and protect the body. They are joined by ligaments and tendons to create a framework to which is attached muscles and soft tissue. As in the human skeleton, there are differences between the equine male and female structure. Female bones are considered generally more slender than those of the male, which are correspondingly larger and heavier, with the female head being proportionally finer. However, the main difference will be found in the shape of the pelvis, the female pelvis being wider to aid the passage of the foal during birth.

The skeleton provides the basis of all movement by providing a stable but mobile structure upon which the muscles can act. It consists of a series of moveable levers supported by ligaments and pulled by muscles. It is not an inert structure devoid of life, instead it is an active organ, which produces blood cells and acts as a reservoir for minerals essential for life.

Bone consists of several layers, a thin membrane known as *periosteum*, which is a specialised connective tissue that covers all bone. This 'bone skin' contains blood vessels and nerves and serves as a point of attachment for muscles, tendons and ligaments by connective tissues fusing with the fibrous layers of the periosteum. The layer beneath, the *periosteal* covering, is a hard dense shell known as *compact or cortical* bone and a mesh-like, spongy structure known as *cancellous* bone. In some bones, there is a central cavity or spaces in the spongy bone, which contains fatty tissue or bone marrow, in which red cells, platelets and most white blood cells are formed. The hard or cortical bone varies in thickness in accordance to the stresses it may have to bear. Hickman and Humphrey (1988) illustrate this feature by pointing out that the large metacarpal, or the *cannon bone* (Fig. 2-16), is thicker dorsally than palmarly and rather more thicker medially than laterally. In essence, bone is thicker and denser where it needs greatest strength.

There are four types of bone, long, short, flat and irregular. Long bones are found in limbs, where they form a system of levers. A long bone is comprised of a shaft and two extremities. Growth occurs at a site between the shaft and the articular surfaces, this is known as the *epiphysis* and this is separated from the bone shaft by the *epiphyseal plate*. The shaft is hollow, with a central cavity known as the *medullary canal* in which is stored the marrow, with the extremities being shaped for articulation. Long bones, according to Henry Gray, are not straight but curved, the curve taking place in two directions, affording the greatest strength to the bone; *Gray's Anatomy* lists the *humerus, radius, ulna, femur, tibia, fibula, metacarpal* and *metatarsal* bones and the phalanges.

Short bones exist where strength and compactness is needed but motion is limited. Where there are a number, they are bound together by ligaments. As examples of this type of bone, Henry Gray lists the carpus and the tarsus but also includes the patellae and the sesamoid bones.

Flat bones are found where protection is needed or a broad surface for the attachment of muscles is required. The list, which Gray sets out, includes the *scapula,* the *sternum,* the *ribs* and the patella.

Irregular bones are defined by their shape and their structure; they too like all other bones, have a covering of periosteum, a layer of compact cortical bone and house a spongy tissue within. The bones within this classification include the *vertebrae* and the *sacrum*.

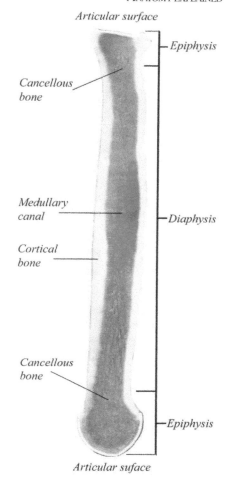

Articular surface

Epiphysis

Cancellous bone

Medullary canal

Diaphysis

Cortical bone

Cancellous bone

Epiphysis

Articular suface

Fig. 2-16: Featured here is a saggital section of the cannon bone, which is a long bone.

Long bones have a shaft or diapysis, which is a tube-like structure that is both strong and rigid. Its central area (the medullary canal, or cavity) is filled with soft yellow bone marrow, while the extremities of the bone, the epiphysis, are composed of spongy bone filled with red bone marrow.

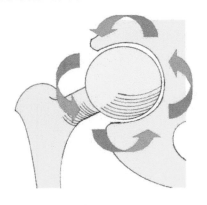

Fig. 2-17: A schematic example of a 'ball and socket' joint.

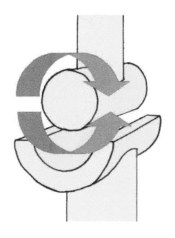

Fig. 2-18: A schematic example of a 'hinge' joint.

JOINTS

Joints, like the bones themselves, are categorised and belong to families, groups or types of joints. Some joints are fixed, like those that can found in the skull; there are also those that allow a little movement, like those of the vertebrae. Where no movement is required, cartilage or connective tissue unites bones. Where the joints are freely moveable, the joint surfaces are covered with articular cartilage, connected by ligaments and lined by a synovial membrane, which secretes synovia or joint fluid.

Within the equine limb, there are fundamentally only two types of joint, *ball and socket joints* (or *enarthrosis* joints) (Fig. 2-17) and *hinge joints* (or *ginglymus* joints) (Fig. 2-18). Both the shoulder and the hip are comprised of enarthrosis joints; these are joints where the distal bone is capable of motion around an infinite number of axes, all of which have one common centre. It is formed by the reception of a sphere-shaped articular surface, which then fits into a cup-like cavity, which is why it is commonly known as a ball and socket joint.

The other type of joint found within the limb is essentially a hinge joint. This type of joint is formed with articular surfaces being shaped to correspond with one another, with those surfaces being held in place by strong lateral ligaments Motion is permitted in one plane only, forwards and backwards; the extent of this motion is considerable. The direction in which the distal bone takes in this motion is never in the same plane as that of the axis of the proximal bone. Furthermore, there is always a certain amount of alteration from the straight line during flexion.

In *Gray's Anatomy*, the classic text on anatomy, the most perfect forms of this type of joint are to be found between the phalanges. Therefore, it is not surprising that in the equine, it is the fetlock, which is considered to be the most perfect example of this type of joint.

MUSCLES, TENDONS AND LIGAMENTS

These soft tissue elements bind together the skeletal framework and act in synchronisation as the nerve endings within the muscles receive impulses from the brain to create motion.

Muscles are composed of bundles of specialised cells, capable of contraction and relaxation and through this motion movement is created. Contraction makes the muscle shorter and draws together the bones to which the muscle is attached; it is through co-ordinated relaxation and contraction that movements of the skeletal frame are accomplished. Skeletal muscles are classified according to the type of action they initiate (Fig. 2-19). An *extensor* will open out a joint whereas a *flexor* will draw the joint together. Skeletal muscles are composed of muscle fibres grouped together to form bundles bound together to form an orderly mass. Small muscles are made up of only a few bundles while larger muscles may be made up of hundreds of bundles. Each fibre is made up of smaller units called myofibrils, which are formed by the microscopic filaments that control contraction. Each muscle fibre is served by a nerve ending, which receives impulses from the brain. The impulses from the brain then set into motion a sequence of electrical and chemical events, which cause the muscle to contract, sensors within the muscles gauge the force of contraction and monitor the stretch, and the brain then assimilates this information in order to limit muscle action.

Tendons are fibrous cords that link muscle to bone and are strong and flexible but are inelastic. They are usually to be found at either end of the muscle belly and are formed from bundles of a white fibrous protein called collagen and contain some blood vessels and nerve endings. The tendons may run in enclosed synovial sheaths which are lubricated by a fluid secreted by the lining of those sheaths, or pass over a synovial bursa, which is a closed sac lined with a synovial membrane containing just a little synovial fluid.

Ligaments are tough bands of white fibrous relatively inelastic tissue that are integral components within the formation of joints, binding bone to bone. However there are some ligaments, which largely contain yellow elastic tissue and it is considered that the elasticity of these ligaments is intended to act as a substitute for muscle power. Four strong distinct ligaments are included within this category and these are called *accessory ligaments*, these ligaments serve as supplementary aids to support the tendons they are associated with and it is one of those accessory ligaments, which can be found in the hip, the accessory femoral ligament that is in fact unique to the equine.

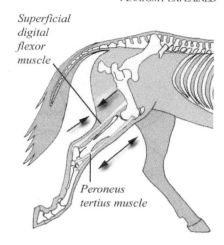

Fig. 2-19: Skeletal muscles work in pairs; where a muscle is placed to pull in one direction there must be a corresponding muscle to pull in the opposite direction. Skeletal muscles are divided into flexors (those that flex a joint) and extensors (those that extend a joint). However, some muscles have dual functions and this is because they may have several attachments.

Illustrated above and part of the reciprocal mechanism of the hindlimb, is the superficial digital flexor muscle; as it contracts the hock is extended. Then as it relaxes and the peroneus tertius muscle simultaneously contracts the hock is flexed.

THE SHOULDER (FORELIMB)

There are considered to be six principal joints within each of the four limbs of the horse. The proximal joints of the foreleg are the shoulder, the elbow and the knee, while in the hind limb there are the hip, the stifle and the hock. The distal joints, those below the knee and the hock, are the fetlock, pastern and pedal.

In the forelimb, the shoulder joint (Fig. 2-20) is formed by the articular cup of the scapula, known as the glenoid cavity, and the articular head of the humerus. The joint is absent of any collateral ligaments to maintain a tight, consistent, functional arrangement between the two bones, instead powerful muscles surround this joint to help keep the bones in place. The *scapula* itself is a broad flat bone with a subtly undulating inner surface, being attached to the trunk of the horse by muscles, ligaments and loose connective tissue. This design allows the scapula a fluid range of movement to glide smoothly over the correspondingly curved surface of the ribcage when pulled by the muscles attached to its surfaces and borders.

Effectively the main body of the horse, the thorax, hangs between the two scapulae positioned on either side of the trunk by muscular attachments. This complex muscular design cradles the suspended thorax within a muscular sling known as the thoracic sling. This

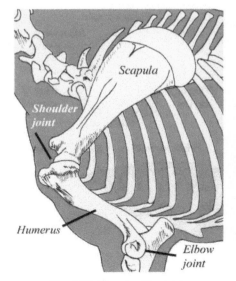

Fig. 2-20: The shoulder joint

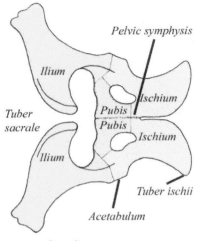

Pelvic symphysis

Ilium

Ischium

Tuber sacrale

Pubis
Pubis

Ilium

Ischium

Tuber ischii

Acetabulum

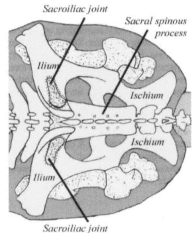

Sacroiliac joint

Sacral spinous process

Ilium

Ischium

Ischium

Ilium

Sacroiliac joint

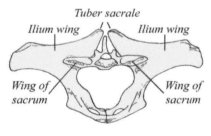

Tuber sacrale

Ilium wing

Ilium wing

Wing of sacrum

Wing of sacrum

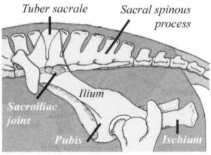

Tuber sacrale

Sacral spinous process

Sacroiliac joint

Ilium

Pubis

Ischium

arrangement provides the body supported between the scapulae with an unparalleled range of movement, which in conjunction with the ball and socket joint of the shoulder, accounts for almost all of the lateral movements executed by the forelimbs during motion.

Lateral movements are those movements where the horse moves forwards and sideways at the same time. These movements occur naturally but in the discipline of dressage are executed upon the command of the rider. Where the limbs move, in an outwards sideways movement, away from the midline of the body, this is called abduction. Where the limbs move in an inward motion, towards, and at times across the midline of the body, this is called adduction.

THE PELVIS (HINDLIMB) (Figs. 2-21-24 - left)

The pelvis is a symmetrical composite bone, made up of two halves with three bones on each side of its wing-like shape, the *ilium*, the *pubis* and the ischium. These three bones begin to fuse together pre-birth and continue to do so while the animal is a foal, with an initial closure at around 10-12 months and total closure being around 4½-5 years. However, in the adult horse it is impossible to identify where they merge into one single structure. In the young animal, the two halves of the pelvic girdle meet through a cartilaginous joint that allows limited movement, which ossifies (converts into bone) through to maturity, and this is called the pelvic *symphysis*. This process begins cranially, moves caudally along the pubis, and extends towards the ischium. This union only measures around 4½-5 inches long (about 11-13 cm) and according to anatomists this connection may not be total, with islands of cartilage remaining even until very late on in life. Dr Deb Bennett, an equestrian and palaeontologist describes the connection of the left and right pubes by saying that they *'are not firmly co-ossified but joined together by short ligaments'*. Dr Bennett goes on to describe the union of the two halves of the pelvic girdle as *'another case of functional Velcro'*. The other case of 'functional Velcro', which she refers to, is the sacroiliac joint and this joint is considered by many to be a common site of potential lameness.

The sacroiliac joints are formed by the attachment of the two halves of the pelvis to the spinal column. On each side of the pelvis, the ilium wing connects to a triangular shaped bone known as the *sacrum*, which consists of five vertebral bones that are fused together pre-birth. It is this connection between the wing of sacrum and the ilium wing that makes up the *sacroiliac joint*. It is considered to have little or no movement; in fact, stability (and not mobility) is desirable within this joint. Researchers who have examined it in detail state that there is little or no joint fluid to be found within it; instead, strong ligaments are the main feature which envelop the joint in order to ensure its stability. Stashak (1987) informs us that since the sacroiliac joint is not meant to be mobile, stresses that produce motion may produce a partial dislocation and that this event is likely to be caused through a cycle of repeated trauma rather than through one single event.

It is worthwhile considering at this juncture that it is the sacroiliac joint which forms the link between limb and spine and that it is these two small areas of attachment that are responsible for the union between the pelvis and the sacral section of the vertebral column. The sacroiliac joint, as small as it is, is the point at which the hind limb, a powerful functioning unit, is joined to the body of the equine.

ASYMMETRY WITHIN THE SHOULDER AND THE PELVIS

Sacroiliac problems are considered a common source of lameness that affects a large number of equines, with body asymmetry often seen as an indication that something is wrong. However, although a singular traumatic injury may be thought to be the origin of such lameness, it should also be considered that the continued repetitive actions of natural behaviour, may themselves lead to an asymmetry and it is possible that those actions may in fact be the root cause of many lamenesses. Therefore, asymmetric behaviour should not just simply be viewed as being the part of any symptom, instead we need to look closely at just what those actions cause in order to decide what adjustments we need to make to the management of those equines who are in our care.

Body-shape and outline needs to be recognised as being something which is influenced by, and adapts to, the frequent and prolonged patterns of stance and movement, with function creating form. Inherent continuous repetitive asymmetric behaviour can, for example, shape the equine's pelvic alignment and if, according to Dr Bennett, the pelvis becomes twisted, then the position of the hip sockets will be affected so that they will no longer lie at equal heights from the ground, with asymmetry of both stance and movement then becoming natural consequences of characterised motion.

In the forelimb, muscle development around the shoulder has also been linked to unlevel action and asymmetric behaviour (Fig. 2-25).

It needs to be remembered that the scapula, a broad flat bone, lies close against the subtle curve of the ribcage but has no bony attachment to it. Instead, it is appended by muscle, ligament and connective tissue.

Different ranges of motion will, as a direct result of usage, create differences in muscle development; a dominant forelimb will create more muscle bulk and functional apparent limb-length differences can be frequently observed, with the dominant leg exhibiting an apparent but measurable shorter distal limb; a phenomenon invariably associated with a broad low-heeled hoof.

Dr Kerry Ridgway DVM, a holistically based veterinarian who has spent many years of his career focusing upon the study of the equine sports performance horse, specializes in muscle tension, imbalance and symmetry and has developed a particular interest in the asymmetries to be found within the body-shape of the horse. Since

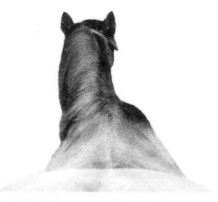

Fig. 2-25: Shoulder and pelvic asymmetry may be found in the majority of horses in a whole range of gradations. It may not be obvious but it is never more obvious than when someone else points it out.

This animal has a 'bulged' right shoulder and a slightly rounder left croup.

It is worth noting that Tony Gonzales, an American farrier, suggested that where a bulging of the shoulder was to be found, it could be frequently observed that the hair at the base of the mane almost invariably fell to the opposite side.

1990, through his daily practice, 90% of his work has been focused upon saddle related problems, shoeing related problems and back pain; this has provided him with the opportunity to study the relationships between the three on a 'first hand basis'. His observations have been found to be intriguing but they have frequently been met with scepticism, so he has continually sought to find better ways to explain his thoughts and the links he has identified, in the hope of creating a greater awareness of what he considers to be a collective pattern of observable occurrences.

Speaking at the *A Bridge to the Future* veterinary conference in 2003, Dr Ridgway presented his paper *Low Heel/High Heel Syndrome*. In his paper he discussed the asymmetries to be found within the shoulders of the horse and catalogued a list of muscles (Fig. 2-26), naming the ***trapezius*** and the ***serratus thoracis*** as being the muscles he considered the most liable to hypertrophy. He also went on to associate these and other well-developed muscles (the ***rhomboids***, the ***deltoids*** and the ***subscapularis***) with the shoulder of a forelimb exhibiting a low-heeled hoof. In contrast, the musculature development of the other limb, which has often been thought of as being atrophied or underdeveloped, he found had often acquired a well-developed ***descending pectoral*** muscle.

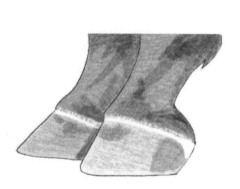

Fig. 2-27: So-called mismatched hooves are where one hoof, within a pair, is considered flatter than the other hoof, which may be considered upright.

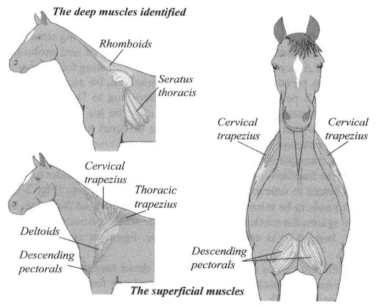

Fig. 2-26: An illustration identifying the muscle groups most liable to hypertrophy.

Dr Ridgway, like a growing number of other authorities, openly makes the link between mismatched hooves (pairs of hooves of differing size and shape) (Fig. 2-27) and the asymmetry of the shoulder region but unlike others, he provides details to give clarity and credence to his interpretation.

So where is all this information leading? Well we all need to think holistically and not think of things in isolation.

The best way to evaluate the horse for shoulder asymmetry is to view it from behind and from a raised vantage point. Depending upon the size of the horse and the height of the observer, a box, stool, or any other sturdy object to stand upon may be required in order to get a better view of the animal's withers and shoulder area. Symmetry is the ideal but in many horses a lateral bulge may be found around the cranial angle of the scapula, this is because the scapula of that particular limb will be placed in a more vertical position.

When the scapula is positioned at an obtuse angle, the **scapulo-humeral** joint (shoulder joint) becomes more extended and effectively creates a vertically longer distance from the point of elbow to the highest point on the withers (fig. 2-28). This opening of the joint also places the point of shoulder in a more caudal position, which according to Dr Ridgway, can be as much as 2 inches further back, when compared with the shoulder of the other limb. In contrast the scapula of the other limb (Fig.2-29), lying in a more flat horizontal plane, will be placed at a more acute angle, with the shoulder joint acquiring a more flexed, or closed attitude, effectively making the proximal limb vertically shorter than its counterpart, thereby creating functional limb-length discrepancies.

The owner or rider does not always notice this disparity between the proximal limbs until saddle-fitting problems are encountered and unlevel actions within the gaits of the horse become a problem.

Saddles, by proportion, are constructed symmetrically, so when placed upon a horse that has developed an asymmetry of the shoulders, the 'bulged' shoulder may strike the edge of the panel as the scapula moves throughout its range of motion (Fig. 2-30). This influence effectively rotates the saddle into a diagonal orientation however this action tends not to provide a similar contact on both sides. The torque, which is created within the tree of the saddle, may unfortunately place excessive pressure upon one side of the thoracic spine that will cause the horse pain and the loss of ability to perform bending and lateral movements.

Minor dissimilarities within the body-shape of the horse may, in themselves, seem fairly innocuous but understanding the cause of any uneven appearance and knowing how best to manage any imbalance is an important part of horsemanship. Prevention is always better than cure and so the realisation that appropriate riding, schooling strategies (corrective exercise) and other alternative therapies that may result in a more evenly balanced horse, should hopefully keep any potential lameness at bay because unfortunately asymmetry means uneven usage, exaggerated usage and damage = lameness.

Although the rider should be the first to notice any asymmetry, frequently it is the farrier who is the first to be aware of its existence and this is hardly surprising. The links that exist between uneven shoulder development; apparent limb-length disparities and hoof size are familiar patterns that the working farrier sees on a daily basis. The general rule is that where there are hooves of different sizes within a pair of limbs, the larger hoof will belong to the limb that will have an effectively shorter distal limb. Where this occurs the proximal limb (from the

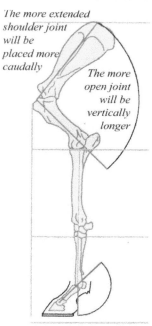

The more extended shoulder joint will be placed more caudally

The more open joint will be vertically longer

The flatter hoofed limb will have a more protracted range of movement.

Fig. 2-28

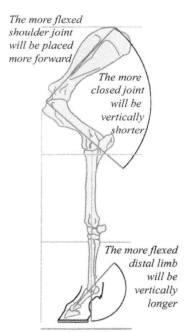

The more flexed shoulder joint will be placed more forward

The more closed joint will be vertically shorter

The more flexed distal limb will be vertically longer

The upright hoofed limb will have a more retracted range of movement

Fig. 2-29

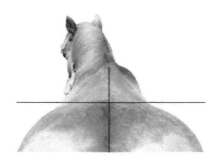

Fig. 2-30: The identification of asymmetries of the shoulder and pelvis may not be as easy as it would seem from this picture but an understanding of how they occur and the implications to the soundness and well-being of the horse and what farriery it will need throughout its life is essential to the management of all equines.

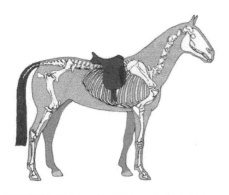

Fig. 2-31: Saddle fitting like farriery is an active part of horse management.

Although in essence saddles are symmetrical, they will be modified to fit the horse for which they are intended and just as the horse's body shape can change so too can the padding within the saddle.

Incorrect saddle fitting can interfere with the shoulder blade, with the front edge of the saddle bumping against the scapular cartilage. This can lead to a shortening of the stride and damage to the latissimus dorsi muscles, which function to draw the limb back under the body when the hoof is on the ground.

elbow up) will be apparently longer (see Fig. 2-28) and from this configuration it can be determined that this limb will be more protractive, achieving a more extended range of movement. The other limb, however, will display a smaller hoof, an apparently longer distal limb and an apparently shorter proximal limb (see Fig. 2-29). This arrangement is consistent with the limb having a more retractive or 'drawn under' range of motion.

So, is there a connection between the asymmetries of the shoulder and those of the pelvis? Well there may be evidence.

Pat Thacker, GPF, RJF, an American farrier, whose interest lies in the promotion of 'Natural Balance' principles and guidelines, conducted a study measuring hoof angles. Through that study, he concluded *'that the great majority of horses do not possess matched angle pairs'*. He also noted that out of the horses within his study group, he was able to make the link that where a fore hoof was found to be steeper than its mate, the diagonally opposite hind hoof was also steeper. He went on to write *'the steep feet occurred 80% of the time on the diagonal [RF, LH or LF, RH]. They occurred 20% of the time on the lateral [RF, RH or LF, LH]'*.

So how does that relate to hind limb asymmetry? Well Tony Gonzales, the legendary farrier from Hawaii, who was probably the first farrier to write about the asymmetries within the equine body, considered it was a 'given' that where a lower heeled hoof was present what he called a 'hunters bump' was also in evidence.

A 'hunters bump' is the phrase given to the visibly noticeable prominence of the ***tuber sacrale***, the part of the pelvis that is positioned at the highest point of each side of the horse's croup. Variations within this area are in fact normal and the appearance of any asymmetry between the two prominences can often be attributed to the amounts of subcutaneous fat and muscle, which shape and cover that particular region, so disparities observed need not always be associated with a bony displacement.

Although what Tony Gonzales viewed as a 'hunters bump' could be challenged, he did link that asymmetry with a low heeled hind hoof, which would seem to coincide with the observations of Pat Thacker. This is because where there is a noticeable muscle development on one shoulder; it is frequently observed that more muscle bulk may be found on the diagonally opposite hind limb (Fig.2-30). So, does this also connect with the observations of Dr Ridgway? Well, in his paper, Dr Ridgway makes a remark about the other diagonal. He noticed that on the diagonal, defined by the forelimb with the high-heeled hoof, should the croup rise more during its motion, then this movement, he thought, would encourage saddle slippage toward the shoulder lacking in muscle (see saddle fitting: Fig. 2-31). However, is this fact or pure conjecture? Here science comes to our aid, Kevin G. Keegan, DVM, MS, Diplomate ACVS, conducted a study into the patterns of pelvic movement in horses. He found that of the horses within his study group, where there was a pelvic asymmetry, whether or not that horse was lame, the total vertical movement of the ***tuber coxae*** was always the greatest on the lower side of the pelvis.

So, are there connections? The evidence is out there, patterns do exist; we just need to join up the dots.

ANATOMY CONTINUED: THE HIP (HINDLIMB)

In the hind limb, lateral movements stem primarily from the hip joint. The hip joint is a ball and socket joint made up from the head of the femur and a deep articular cup named the ***acetabulum***, which is formed by the three pelvic bones, the ***ilium***, the ***pubis*** and the ***ischium***. The joint permits movement in every direction although it is considered that its ability to abduct, or to move outward away from the midline of the body, is limited because of the joint's ***accessory femoral ligament***. One end of the accessory femoral ligament, which is unique to the horse, synthesises with the ***prepubic tendon*** of the opposite side, which is attached to the ***rectus abdominis muscle***. The other end passes through a groove cut into the rim of the acetabulum, known as the ***acetabular notch***, to become attached to a corresponding non-articular notch on the head of the femur, which is then held in place by the ***transverse acetabular ligament***. It is through this arrangement that, according to Dr Bennett, as *'the rectus abdominis contracts, the femoral head is rotated inward and thus the stifle outward'*. Dr Bennett also states that as the hind limb takes in a forward motion, an accompanying rotation takes place aligning the stifle outwards and the hock inwards. Smythe & Goody also make this same point by stating that as the hip is flexed an outward rotation of the femur occurs (Fig. 2-32). So, what does this motion mean to the farrier? Bennett goes on to explain, in her opinion, any trim or appliance which seeks to block this normal outward rotation of the hind limb, either in stance or motion will, in fact, prove to be detrimental to all the joints of the limb.

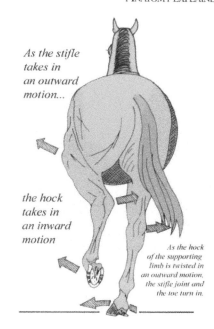

As the stifle takes in an outward motion...

the hock takes in an inward motion

As the hock of the supporting limb is twisted in an outward motion, the stifle joint and the toe turn in.

Fig. 2-32: During the protraction of the hindlimb, a series of reciprocal motions take place; as the hip is flexed, the stifle takes in an outward motion, while the hock takes in an inward motion.

An opposite affect can be noted in the supporting hindlimb during retraction.

THE JOINTS BELOW THE SHOULDER AND THE HIP

It is from the ball and socket joints of the shoulder and hips that the vast majority of all medial and lateral motion originates. In the forelimb, the distal aspect of the scapula and the proximal articular head of the humerus form the shoulder joint (Fig. 2-33). The joint below is that of the ***elbow***, which takes its form from the distal surface of the humerus, the surface of which is shaped for articulation with the ***radius*** and the ***ulna***.

The shape of the distal end of the humerus is created by an oblique groove separating two smooth prominent ***condyles***, the medial one being the larger. Its shape is considered to permit motion in one plane only without any free lateral movement. However, its design does bring about a controlled range of motion, according to Smythe & Goody, during flexion *'the bones of the forearm (radius and ulna) do not move in the exact plane of the humerus, but rotate a little outwards around the anatomical axis of the radius'*. This controlled range of lateral motion is in fact indicative of the type of joint that is commonly labelled as belonging to the classified family of ginglymus joints.

Ginglymus joints have the unparalleled and identifiable feature of having a three-dimensional range of motion with the distal bones

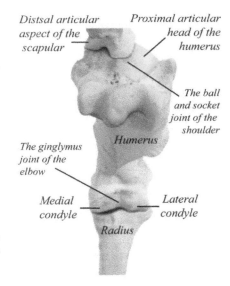

Distsal articular aspect of the scapular

Proximal articular head of the humerus

The ball and socket joint of the shoulder

Humerus

The ginglymus joint of the elbow

Medial condyle

Lateral condyle

Radius

Fig. 2-33: An anterior view of the shoulder and elbow joints.

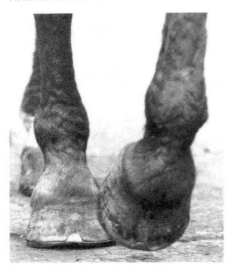

Fig. 2-34: Breakover occurs, almost without exception, at the lateral aspect of the toe. Attempts at 'correcting' the breakover could create torsional stress related injuries (Photo: J Watts).

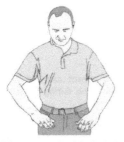

Elbows out, hands face in.

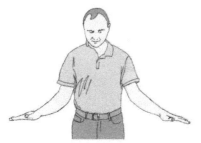

Elbows in, hands turn out.

Fig. 2-35: A simple demonstration can help us understand how the positioning of the elbow can create a toe-in or a toe-out conformation (based on an idea of Dr Bennett's).

and the proximal bones never sharing the same axis. This unique feature of all ginglymus joints is without doubt the major obstacle when it comes to an honest appreciation of any limb's joint mechanics. The failure to accept how unique and complex each limb actually is, provides through continued ignorance, a potential cause of discomfort and the possible cause of lameness to many equines. Farriery is too often sold as a means of 'correction' with attempts at altering conformation to improve the flight of the hoof and limb in the mature horse, having the potential to cause damage. Dr Hilary Clayton touches upon this subject when discussing the differences between '*static hoof balancing*', where an assessment is made of the limb at stance and '*dynamic hoof balancing*', where an assessment is made of the limb during motion.

In mediolateral hoof balancing, adjustments can be made to the heights of the medial and lateral hoof wall. The skilful farrier will not merely be trimming to reduce horn growth but will also be aiming to optimise the weight bearing functions of the hoof, facilitate breakover and assist in the achievement of a straight flight pattern during the swing phase of motion. However, by seeking to alter the natural breakover of the limb in order to produce a breakover at the centre of the toe, with the belief of producing a straighter arc in flight, could in fact create torsional forces within the hoof and limb (Fig. 2-34).

Colloquial phrases are often used to describe the deviations from the straight, dishing, paddling; plaiting and winging are all used to describe the many variants of *abduction* and *adduction*. Abduction is when the limbs move in an outwards sideways motion, adduction is where the limbs move in an inward sideways motion. Dr Clayton established that the wear pattern of the hoof or shoe at the toe was a good indicator of the preferred side of breakover. It was also found that if the horse was shod to facilitate the breakover at the preferred location, then there was often a marked reduction in the amount of winging or plaiting.

Determining the direction each joint faces and then trying to analyse its unique range of movement and understand how those elements influence the form and function of the limb as a whole, may prove difficult if not elusive. However, with regard to the positioning of the elbow, Dr Bennett states the direction it faces is the principal determinate factor that then affects the set of the forelimb, so governing whether the horse will be described as having a toe-in or toe-out conformation. A simple demonstration can help us understand this more easily. When we move our elbows away from our body our hands turn in and when we bring our elbows close to our body, our hands turn out (Fig. 2-35). Dr Goody adds further to our understanding of how the elbow affects form and function and reports that the mechanics of this ginglymus joint are such that the elbow may in fact produce some dishing (abduction) during elbow flexion especially during trot. So by looking at this one joint alone, not in isolation but as part of the limb functioning as a unit, it begs the question, in the mature horse, should attempts be made to alter conformation and breakover, when the limb is primarily made up of ginglymus joints?

THE STIFLE JOINT (HINDLIMB)

The *stifle* in the horse can be compared to the ***human knee*** with the ***gaskin*** akin to the ***human calf*** and the ***hock*** analogous with the ***human ankle***. The stifle joint, which is the largest joint in the body, is sometimes referred to as the true knee and is generally considered to be both complex and prone to injury. It occupies the equivalent position in the hindlimb, as does the elbow in the forelimb. The joint itself is a composite joint made up of two separate articulations, the ***femorotibial articulation*** made up of the *tibia* and *femur* and the ***femoropatellar articulation*** made up of the ***patella*** and the ***femur***. The overall product of these two articulations is the creation of a single hinge or ginglymus joint.

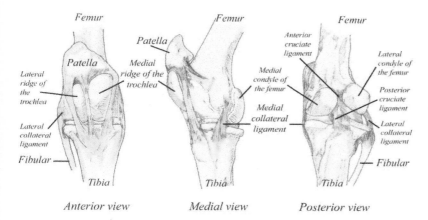

Anterior view   Medial view   Posterior view

Fig. 2-36: The stifle joint

Just as in the human knee, there is a kneecap (the patella), a small flat bone, which rides within the obliquely set articular condyles of the distal surface of the femur (*the femoral trochlea*). The patella is a *sesamoid* bone and the largest of its type; other sesamoids can be found at the *fetlock joint* and the *pedal joint*. Sesamoids are, according to Dr Bennett, *intra-tendinal bursae*, which have become ossified (converted into bone). Intra-tendinal bursae are thick *fibro-cartilaginous* pads, which have been developed within the tendon of a muscle and are not true bone. They tend to occur where a tendon must pass around a sharp bend and function as a dampening feature to protect the inner aspect of the tendon by both diminishing the friction and modifying the pressure upon the tendon from which it originates. They may also serve to multiply the force and reduce the effort required by the muscle to fulfil its designated task.

    The stifle has an organised assembly of ligaments that maintain a structural stability. There are medial and lateral collateral ligaments that are there to limit lateral movement and there are cruciate ligaments that cross each other resembling the letter X, again these are in place to provide stability.

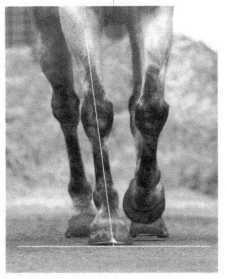

Fig. 2-37: It is normal for supporting limbs during progression to be positioned at an angle of around 84°-86°. Therefore, lateral heel landing should be considered normal (Photo: J Watts).

THE RADIUS AND THE ULNA (FORELIMB)

The radius and the ulna combine together to create the forearm of the animal. In the horse, the radius is the larger of the two bones and unlike in the human, these two bones are joined together. In the young animal, they are united by ligamentous fibres, which become ossified as the horse matures, so unlike in the human there is no movement between the radius and the ulna. In the human, these two bones run parallel but do not touch except at their ends, with the proximal end of the radius being designed to roll against the shaft of the ulna. This arrangement allows the human hands to adjust their orientation, freely enabling the palm of the hand to be turned upwards (*supinate*) or downwards (*pronate*). However, in the horse these two bones are fused together both proximally and distally, which is why, as Dr Bennett states, their union '*totally precludes rotary motion of any kind within this segment of the limb*'. So, as the design of the joints within the equine limb are predominantly ginglymus, when the limb is extended prior to ground contact during the period of **retraction** and deceleration, the initial contact will be determined by a fixed skeletal positioning. Therefore, during motion with the body of the equine facing the line of progression it is normal for the limb to contact the ground at an angle of around 84°-86° (Fig. 2-37). This occurs because during forward motion (*protraction*) the hoof is positioned close to the line of progression in order to support the equine's centre of mass to maintain the equine's equilibrium. It is this action, known as convergence, which determines the normality of the lateral heel landing first.

THE TIBIA AND FIBULA (HINDLIMB)

In the hindlimb, the tibia and fibula combine to form that part of the limb known as the gaskin, which is situated between the stifle and the hock joints. As with the radius and the ulna in the forelimb, the tibia and fibula become fused with age creating a similar functional parallel, ensuring that no rotational movement can take place within that portion of the limb. However, because of the relationship between the proximal joint, the stifle, the distal joint and the hock, a rotation does appear to take place and this occurs because both joints are ginglymus joints. O.R. Adams, author of the classic text *Lameness in Horses*, noted this action and wrote, '*As the body weight passes over the hind limb, it is not uncommon to observe a considerable outward twist of the hock joint...at the same time, the stifle joint and the toe turn in*' (Fig. 2-38). This action is normal; Dr Bennett recognises this and adds further to the evidence by stating that during hind limb protraction the stifle is rotated outward and the hock inward. This movement is often echoed in the wear pattern of hind shoes; it is not unusual to identify more wear occurring to the lateral branches of each shoe, with the greatest wear taking place to the lateral branch of the dominant hind.

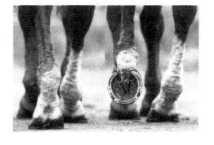

Fig. 2-38: As the body weight passes over the supporting hindlimb, it is not unusual to see an outward twist of the hock, creating an inward twisting of the hoof, frequently resulting in an increased wear pattern to the lateral branch of the hoof or shoe (Photo: J Watts).

THE CARPUS OR KNEE (FORELIMB)

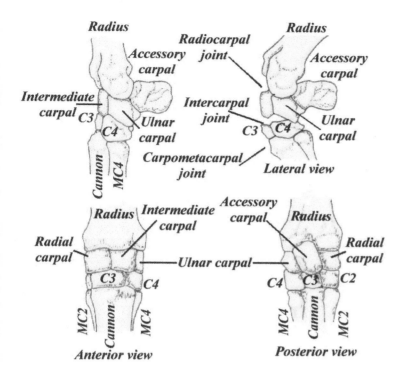

Fig. 2-39: The carpus or the knee joint.

The first carpal bone (C1) that may be found embedded within the medial collateral ligament is frequently absent and so is omitted from this illustration.

The knee, which is a homologue of our wrist, mainly acts as a hinge joint supported by collateral ligaments. It is frequently described as having seven or eight bones arranged in two rows, one above the other. The *radial*, the *intermediate*, the *ulnar* and the *accessory* carpal bones form the proximal row, while the *first; second, third* and *fourth* carpal bones form the distal row. When the foot is raised close to the elbow, the joint can be seen to be a compound joint with a gap becoming noticeable between the radius and the proximal row of bones (*the radio-carpal joint*). A second space is also noticeable which forms between the two rows of carpal bones (*the intercarpal joint*) and a third (but negligible) gap is also present between the distal row of carpal bones and the metacarpus (*the carpometacarpal joint*). Collectively, these three joints form the carpus or knee. Although the carpometacarpal joint is considered a plane joint, the knee as a unit is considered to be another example of a ginglymus joint, having motion in one plane, flexion and extension. However, during its movement, some abduction and adduction may be noted but this is because as with all ginglymus joints it is more complex than a conventional door hinge and should be considered three-dimensional.

THE TARSUS OR HOCK (HINDLIMB)

The *hock*, which is comparable to the *human ankle*, is another joint similar to that of the knee in that it is actually considered to consist of three joints, although it is only through one of those joints, the *tibiotarsal or tarsocural joint*, that the hock takes in its motion. The other joints which make up this complex compound joint are bound together by strong ligaments and are thought to play no part in its general movement, although some minute displacement of the bones may exist between them.

The hock joint is another example of a ginglymus joint, having a great range of unidirectional movement. It is considered to be one of the most complex joints in the horse and, according to Dr Hilary Clayton, its functions are to absorb energy, provide propulsion and act to raise and lower the height of the hoof during the swing phase.

There are six bones that make up the tarsus and they are arranged in three rows tightly bound together by ligaments. The proximal row consists of the *talus* (also known as the *tibial tarsal* bone or, the *astragalus*) and the *calcaneus*. In the middle row, which is primarily made up of one single bone, is the *central tarsal (TC)* and in the distal row, there are the *first and second tarsals (T1+2)*, which are fused together, and the *third tarsal (T3)*. The *fourth tarsal (T4)*, a six-sided bone, occupies both part of the distal and middle rows and is positioned directly beneath the calcaneus bone.

Fig. 2-40: The hock joint (after Wyn-Jones, 1988).

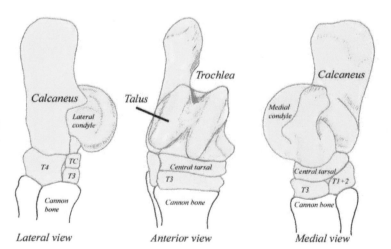

Lateral view   Anterior view   Medial view

It is the striking and identifiable shape of the articular surfaces of the proximal bones that provide the hock with a controlled three-dimensional range of motion. The *talus* has a pulley-shaped articular surface known as the *trochlea*, which is set at an oblique angle to the long axis of the limb, around which the *cochlear* surface of the tibia spirals about. The design supplies the joint with a synchronism of motion that initiates an outward rotation of the limb as the hock joint flexes. This complex sequential action takes place at the same time as the other joints within the limbs fulfil their roles. It is the synchronicity of the organised movements between the joints and the limbs that permits the placement of the hooves beneath the midline of the animal during progression. It is the same complex design of each joint acting within the unit of the limb that also allows the non-supporting limbs to be carried away from the supporting limbs to avoid interference and these actions are the functions and qualities of the ginglymus joint.

THE BONES BELOW THE KNEE AND HOCK

The distal row of carpal bones rests upon the proximal ends of the *large or third metacarpal*, commonly known as the *cannon bone* and the medial and lateral *small metacarpals*, the *second* and *fourth metacarpals*, commonly known as the *splint bones*. The positioning and order of these three bones should not be too difficult to remember when thinking in terms of comparative anatomy. The second metacarpal is representative of our second finger (the one next to our thumb), while our third finger is akin to the phalanges of the equine digit; the horse effectively stands upon its middle finger. Similarly, the fourth metacarpal is not too difficult to remember because it shares the same relative positioning of our fourth finger and is to be found on the outer or lateral side of the limb.

The splint bones are attached to the shaft of the large metacarpal by short ligamentous fibres (*the interosseous ligament*); this union being another case of what Dr Bennett describes as 'functional Velcro'. The bones of the metacarpus, the second, third and fourth metacarpals function as a single unit, providing support to the knee. However, because the third metacarpal or cannon bone is itself supported by the column of bones known as the phalanges and the splint bones are unsupported, that 'functional Velcro' described by Dr Bennett can at times become damaged.

SPLINTS

The fourth carpal bone rests upon the fourth metacarpal and the lateral aspect of the top or proximal articular surface of the cannon or third metacarpal. The third carpal bone rests upon the third or large metacarpal (the cannon) but also finds some added support given by the second metacarpal (the medial splint bone). However, it is the second carpal bone, which singularly supports the medial or second metacarpal along with the entire weight it has to bear. It is considered that this arrangement lends the medial splint more vulnerable to damage created by force, compression and torque than the lateral splint. Therefore, splints are more commonly found at the site of union between the second and third metacarpals, on the medial aspect of the

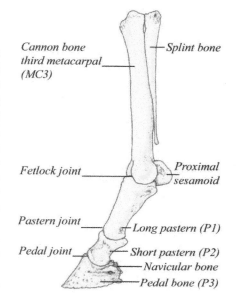

Cannon bone third metacarpal (MC3)

Splint bone

Fetlock joint

Proximal sesamoid

Pastern joint

Long pastern (P1)

Pedal joint

Short pastern (P2)

Navicular bone

Pedal bone (P3)

Fig. 2-41: The bones below the knee and hock.

In the hindlimb the cannon and splint bones are considerably longer than those of the forelimb and share similar respective positions but are named the second, third and fourth metatarsals.

The digital bones however, are slightly smaller in shape than those of the forelimb and are similarly named (after Emery, Miller and Van Hoosen, 1977).

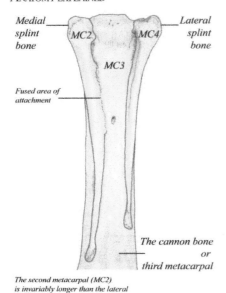

Medial splint bone

Lateral splint bone

MC2

MC4

MC3

Fused area of attachment

The cannon bone or third metacarpal

The second metacarpal (MC2) is invariably longer than the lateral

Fig. 2-42: The metacarpal bones.

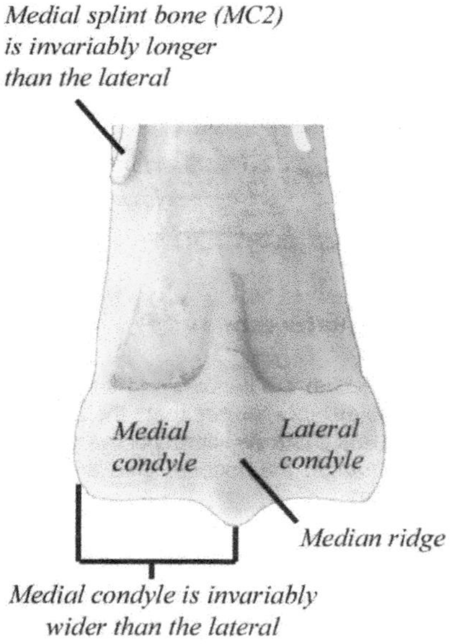

Medial splint bone (MC2) is invariably longer than the lateral

Medial condyle

Lateral condyle

Median ridge

Medial condyle is invariably wider than the lateral

Fig. 2-43: The distal articular surface of the third metacarpal.

cannon rather than on the lateral aspect between the third and fourth metacarpals.

Splints occur as the result of the fibrous attachments between the splint bones and the cannon becoming torn. An inflammatory reaction takes place in the periosteal covering (the membrane that covers the bone), resulting in the ossification of the tissue surrounding the damaged area. Splints can develop in all horses of all ages but this type of injury is more associated with young stock up to around six years of age. The most common site of this type of injury is being the medial splint in the forelimb. Hindlimbs can also be affected but when this occurs there is preponderance towards the lateral splint being the most prone to this type of injury. Splints rarely cause a problem once they are formed but the horse is generally rested when they first occur. In the mature horse, this type of injury is less of a problem because as the horse gets older the splint bones generally become solidly fused to the cannon.

THE FETLOCK

The cannon bone is the main bone positioned between the knee and the fetlock; attached to the cannon bone on both sides, are the medial or lateral splint bones, the medial one being the larger. The two splint bones form a channel in which the ***suspensory ligament*** lies. At the distal end of the bone is the joint known as the ***fetlock***. This joint has been described as a perfect ginglymus joint and its design holds the key to understanding just how complex the limb actually is.

The fetlock, also known as the ***metacarpophalangeal*** joint, is a ginglymus joint which has such a clear and definite construction that it provides a good opportunity for students and interested parties to grasp the fundamental properties of this type of joint. It has a range of motion frequently assumed to be limited to simple flexion and extension; however, its form in shape and structure belies its seemingly singular motion and provides it with an illusive but controlled action. During the progression of locomotion this joint is subject to the greatest stress of any joint within the limb and this is because at times the animal's entire body-weight may be bearing down upon a single supporting fetlock. To support and maintain stability the articular surface at the distal extremity of the cannon bone features a bony ridge, which slots into a corresponding groove shaped within the proximal articular surface of the ***long pastern***, otherwise known as the ***proximal phalanx, first phalanx,*** or ***P1***. It is because of this rigid design that it is assumed by some authorities that this arrangement prevents the joint from rotating from side to side and from left to right and that ginglymus joints compromise the horse's ability to compensate for any foot imbalance. This line of thought has also led those same authorities to think that this type of joint does not allow a complete range of motion which can then adapt to uneven loading. The idea that ginglymus joints are like door hinges is naïve and it is disconcerting that there are those who think of them in such a way.

Whilst all free abduction and adduction originates from the shoulder and the hip, controlled medial and lateral motion within the limb is addressed within the complex design of ginglymus joints, which are all set at a camber with one another.

The bones that make up the fetlock joint are the distal end of the cannon bone, which forms a profile to transmit a controlled range of motion, and the proximal end of the long pastern, which acts as a reciprocating follower. Two other bones feature within the joint and they are known as the *proximal sesamoids*.

At the distal end of the cannon bone, there is a central ridge, known as the *median ridge* or *saggital ridge*. This central ridge is located between two irregular oval shaped facets known as the *medial* and *lateral condyles*, the medial condyle being shorter and squatter, presenting a wider articular surface and the lateral condyle presenting a narrower, smaller articular surface. It is this dynamic design which ensures that the proximal bone and the distal bone never take in the same range of motion but more importantly, while the joint flexes and extends, medial and lateral motions simultaneously occur. As the fetlock extends under weight-bearing this design allows the joint to descend medially allowing the cannon to position itself at an angle with the ground surface and maintain the hoof's supportive position under the equine's body mass.

The two proximal sesamoid bones incorporated within this joint are pyramidal in shape and are bound together by the *intersesamoidean ligament*, or *palmar ligament*, which forms a passageway for the digital flexor tendons. These irregular shaped bones are an integral feature of the *suspensory ligament* otherwise known as the *interosseous* or the *superior sesamoidean ligament* and rather than being true bone are considered ossified bursae, a bursa being a small fluid-filled saclike cavity found in tissue where friction would otherwise occur. An intra-tendinal bursa is a thick fibro-cartilaginous pad, which develops within the tendon of a muscle. In the horse, the suspensory ligament is the anatomical equivalent of the *medial interosseous muscle,* which is present in all other animals that have more than one toe. Through the evolutionary process of the horse, this muscle has been reduced to tendon fibres, although individual horses within some breeds still retain a small proportion of muscle fibres.

The suspensory ligament, which originates from the distal row of carpal bones and the palmar proximal extremity of the cannon bone, follows the channel formed by the medial and lateral splint bones. At the distal extremity of the cannon it divides into two branches, which unite with the medial and lateral sesamoids, each branch then continues downwards and forwards to the dorsal surface of the *proximal phalanx*, or *first phalanx (P1)*, commonly known as the *long pastern*, there it joins the common digital extensor tendon.

The sesamoids, defined as the medial and lateral proximal sesamoids, are situated with the dorsal surfaces lying against the respective condyles of the cannon bone. However, when the joint is fully flexed the sesamoids lose contact with the condyles and ride up over the back of the cannon but bone-to-bone contact is prevented here by the presence of ligament.

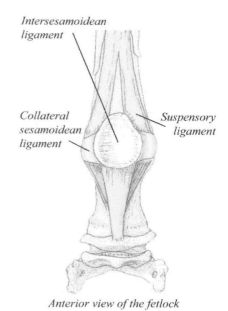

Anterior view of the fetlock

Figs. 2-44: The fetlock joint (after Emery, Miller and Van Hoosen, 1977).

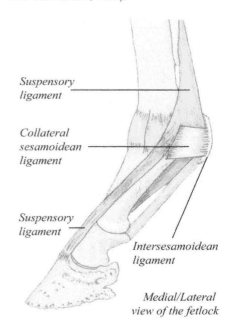

Medial/Lateral view of the fetlock

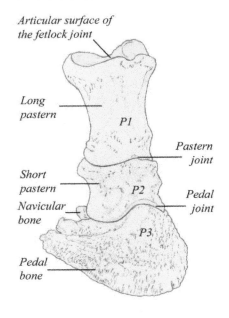

Articular surface of
the fetlock joint

Long
pastern

P1

Pastern
joint

Short
pastern

P2

Pedal
joint

Navicular
bone

P3

Pedal
bone

Figs. 2-45: The bones below the fetlock
(Freeman, 1796).

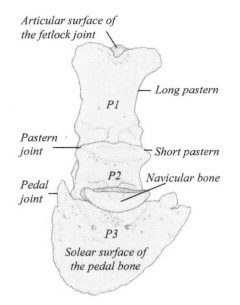

Articular surface of
the fetlock joint

P1

Long pastern

Pastern
joint

Short pastern

P2

Navicular bone

Pedal
joint

P3

Solear surface of
the pedal bone

THE BONES BELOW THE FETLOCK

There are three main bones below the fetlock and they can be compared to the bones which make up fingers. They are called the phalanges, the first phalanx (P1), the second phalanx (P2) and the third phalanx (P3). Like all the other bones, they too have a range of other common names.

The proximal bone (P1), which forms the distal part of the fetlock joint, is known as the long pastern (in old texts *os suffraginis*). Its proximal articular surface is shaped to receive the distal articular surface of the cannon bone and to act as a reciprocating follower. The distal end of the long pastern is shaped to fit into the proximal articular surface of the short pastern, or middle phalanx (P2) (in old texts referred to as the *os coronae*). These two bones create the joint, which is commonly known as the pastern joint.

The pastern joint (proximal interphalangeal joint) is created by these short, strong, robust bones that provide various attachment sites for the flexor and extensor tendons. The pastern joint is similar to that of the fetlock in that it is another ginglymus joint. However, the joint is fairly restrictive and considered to be totally rigid when fully extended.

The pedal joint or distal interphalangeal joint, is housed entirely within the hoof and is sometimes referred to as the coffin joint.

The distal articular surface of the short pastern and the articular surface of the pedal bone (*os pedis*) also referred to as the third phalanx (P3), create the joint. However there is also the distal sesamoid or navicular bone present, which helps to facilitate fluid movement by creating less friction by providing a relatively smooth surface where the deep digital flexor tendon passes over the joint

TENDONS AND ACCOMPANYING MUSCLES OF THE LOWER FORE AND HIND LIMBS

Controlling and supporting each lower limb there are two extensor tendons and two flexor tendons (Fig. 2-46). The ***common digital extensor tendon*** continues down from the ***common extensor muscle***, which has attachments to the distal region of the humerus and the proximal region of the radius. It runs down the front of the cannon, the fetlock joint, and the phalanges to attach itself to the apex (***extensor process***) of the pedal bone (***distal phalanx***). As it passes down the front of the ***first and second phalanx,*** (the long and short pasterns) it sends out attachments to the proximal regions of both bones and it is between these two sites of attachment that the tendon's width becomes greatly increased. At about halfway down the front of the long pastern, the tendon is united with the ***medial*** and ***lateral extensor branches*** of the ***suspensory ligament,*** there the two branches of the suspensory ligament and the tendon merge into one.

The *lateral digital extensor muscle* originates from the proximal region of the humerus with additional attachments to the ulna and the lateral-proximal aspect of the radius. The main tendon of this muscle the *lateral digital extensor tendon* passes down the dorso-lateral surface of the cannon bone and over the front of the fetlock joint to become attached to the proximal aspect of the long pastern (the first phalanx).

The *superficial digital flexor tendon (SDFT)* is a furtherance of the *superficial digital flexor muscle,* which originates from the distal extremity of the humerus. Above the knee the tendon is joined by a wide fibrous band that is anchored to the distal half of the radius, this is the tendons' *accessory ligament*, which is also termed the *superior check ligament*. The tendon passes down the palmar aspect of the cannon, both covering and in unison with the *deep digital flexor tendon (DDFT)*. At the fetlock joint it widens and encircles the DDFT forming a collar, or ring, through which the DDFT passes, both tendons are then held close to the joint by a ligament known as the *palmar annular ligament.* The superficial tendon divides, or bifurcates, about midway down the pastern, the two branches are then attached distally to the first phalanx and proximally to the second phalanx, also at this point, the two tendons (the SDFT and the DDFT) are held in place by the *proximal annular ligament*.

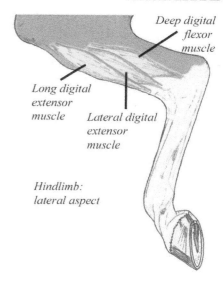

Fig. 2-46: The digital muscles of the hindlimb. The positioning of the superficial digital flexor muscle can be seen in fig. 2-19.

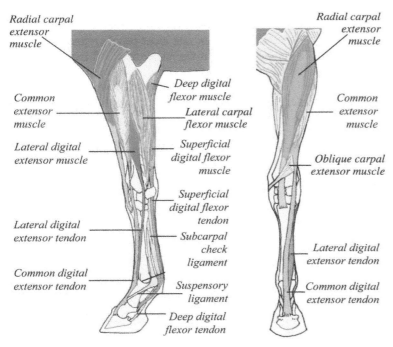

Fig. 2-47: The tendons and accompanying muscles of the lower forelimb.

The ***deep digital flexor muscle*** originates from the distal extremity of the humerus, the proximal extremity of the ulna and the palmar surface of the radius. Down the back of the cannon, the tendon is positioned between the superficial digital flexor tendon and the suspensory ligament. At about half-way down the back of the cannon the deep digital tendon is joined by an accessory ligament known as the ***inferior, or subcarpal, check ligament***, which is a continuation of the ***palmar carpal ligament***. The check ligament assists the flexor tendon and is considered to be the supporting agent, which allows the horse to sleep whilst standing up.

After the superficial digital tendon divides, the deep digital tendon continues its path being held in position by the ***distal annular ligament***. Becoming broader, it passes over the navicular bone and fans out to become attached to the solear surface of the pedal bone, at a point known as the semilunar crest. Where the tendon passes over the navicular bone, or distal sesamoid, there is a bursa, a fluid-filled area to facilitate gliding and reduce friction. The role of the navicular area is to protect the tendon and to dissipate force but also to increase the effective leverage and power of the muscle. However, hyperextension of the pedal joint caused through inadequate farriery can lead to excessive strain and over taxation of the general area, the resulting lameness often labelled as navicular syndrome.

THE VASCULAR SUPPLY AND NERVOUS SYSTEM TO THE HORSE'S FOOT

Possibly the fundamental element that most people remember about these aspects of anatomy is that if the farrier trims off too much horn the hoof will bleed and where there is blood there is likely to be associated pain. However, that is a rather limited summing up of what is a very complex and integral aspect of farriery; there is more to it than that.

The heart and blood vessels exist to provide a continuous flow of blood around the body to deliver the tissues with oxygen and life giving nutrients; the system also removes waste products such as carbon dioxide. Arteries carry the blood all over the body branching out into smaller arteries known as arterioles and these in turn branch further into extremely fine vessels known as capillaries. These tiny blood vessels have thin walls, which allow oxygen and other nutrients to pass easily from the blood into the tissues while other waste products are allowed to pass in the opposite direction. The de-oxygenated blood is carried from the capillaries into small veins known as venules, which in turn join to form veins that return the blood to the heart.

The blood supply to the horse's foot is provided through the ***medial*** and ***lateral digital arteries***, these branches having been formed by the bifurcation of the ***medial common palmar digital artery***, this occurs three quarters of the way down the cannon bone just above the fetlock joint. The digital arteries then diverge, descending distally

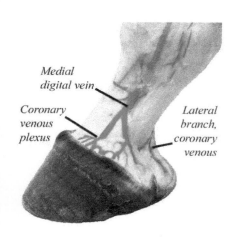

Medial digital vein

Coronary venous plexus

Lateral branch, coronary venous

Fig. 2-48: The medial view of a morbid specimen with the skin removed.

passing either side of the fetlock around the outer surfaces of the sesamoid bones and continue downwards parallel to the borders of the deep flexor tendon. As each digital artery descends, it divides and then subdivides creating a highly complex vascular network, serving to supply nutrition to all the sensitive tissue within the hoof. When they reach the ***third or distal phalanx*** (***pedal bone***), they enter the **solear foramen**, a passageway within the bone, which allows them to unite creating that which is known as the ***terminal arch***. There they subdivide spreading branches throughout the **pedal bone**, extending to the ***sensitive laminae*** and the ***sensitive sole***, forming the artery around the circumference of the bone known as the ***circumflex artery***.

De-oxygenated blood is carried back to the heart and lungs through a similar network of small veins. The ***circumflex vein*** runs parallel to the circumflex artery and blood from this vein is dispersed via an intersecting arrangement of communicating vessels known as the ***solear venous plexus***. There are a number of venous plexuses within the hoof where the blood is gathered and dispersed as it continues with its return journey to be reprocessed, stored or re-entered into general circulation. On its journey from the heart to the tissues, blood is forced through the arteries at a high pressure. However, on its return, the blood is at a low pressure and is kept moving by the muscles in the limbs compressing the walls in the veins and by valves preventing the blood from flowing backwards. It is considered the venous plexuses are areas where the blood gathers within the hoof before the pressure of weight bearing helps effect a venous return from the digit. When the foot takes weight, blood pressure is raised and the veins are emptied and when the foot is raised, the pressure is reduced and the veins fill. This vascular arrangement has also been thought to contribute to the hoof's functions by acting as a kind of dampening hydraulic system to help reduce concussion.

The nerves of the leg and hoof follow similar pathways, as do the arteries and veins. The nervous system gathers information to relay to the brain and forms a pathway to transmit commands from the brain to the far reaches of the body (***peripheral nerves***). The central processing unit responsible for organising such a major task is known as the ***central nervous system***, comprising the brain and the spinal cord. Input of information comes from the sense organs and output (***motor***) instructions go to the skeletal muscles, internal organs and glands. A labyrinth of organised connecting cables fan out from the central nervous system, these cables, which relay information, are the nerves, each nerve is made up from a bundle of axons. It is along these axons that electrical impulses are transmitted directing information and creating a chain of command. Some nerves carry only sensory fibres and some only motor fibres but most carry both. Sensory fibres carry information to the central nervous system from the receptors located at the nerve ends while others have a motor function carrying instructions from the central nervous system to muscles and glands.

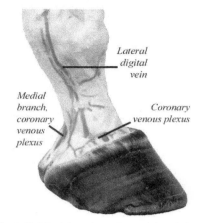

Fig. 2-49: The lateral view of a morbid specimen with the skin removed.

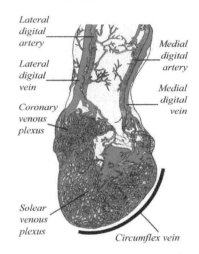

Figs. 2-50: The venous system of the digit (Freeman, 1796).

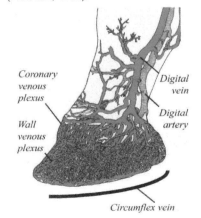

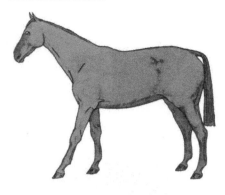

Fig. 2-51: The 'pointing' stance (after W.S. Codrington 1974). After a long-term lameness, the hoof of the sound limb can widen and flatten.

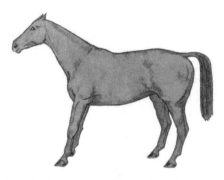

Fig. 2-52: The 'laminitic' stance (after W.S. Codrington 1974). Although the horse attempts to take weight off the toe, heel height increases. As the horse moves, a heel first motion is normal.

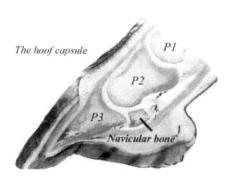

The hoof capsule P1

P2

P3

Navicular bone

Fig. 2-53: A saggital section of the hoof. (Photo supplied by Samuel Beeley, farrier, UK).

PROPRIOCEPTION

Information can be collected and responses made about the body's relative position to the world around it, causing adjustments to be made to both posture and balance through the contraction of muscles and this is called *proprioception*. Sensory nerve endings are located within muscles, tendons, joints and sensory hair cells within the inner ear and these are called *proprioceptors*. During movement, there is a continuous feedback and update of information from the proprioceptors within the limbs and body as well as from the eyes and it is this flow of information that helps ensure smooth actions and co-ordination. Although reactions occur far quicker from information received from receptors imbedded in joints, tendons and muscles, the most prevalent of all the information feedback is received from the horse's eyes.

The hoof and limb is full of sensors relaying a constant stream of information about the environment, the contact between the ground and hoof and the positioning of the limb. During motion, this information then 'tells' the body to organise itself according to the conditions and speed at which it is travelling. During stance, the mechanism is the same with the ability of the self-regulation of posture through movement to maintain balance. The foot at times becomes the influential sensor and at others, the arrangement of the joints, relative to their spatial location, affects the positioning of the limb.

Pain influences stance and motion, likewise stance and motion influences hoof and body-shape. Examples of this can be found in animals with a history of lameness, with a smaller hoof being associated with lameness or unevenness of gait (Fig. 2-51). Horses with laminitis, a condition affecting the union between bone and hoof wall, can be seen making great efforts to keep most of their bodyweight behind their painful toes, and hoof shape itself can also affect well-balanced movement (Fig. 2-52). As stance and the positioning of the centre of mass primarily influence hoof shape and arrangements of the limbs, primarily control motion, how the hoof makes contact with the ground during progression may be more due to skeletal positioning than hoof shape. However, poor farriery, failure to redress and maintain the hoof's correct balance, will lead to lameness because poorly managed hooves can literally send shock waves and disturbances throughout the equine's body.

THE HOOF

The hoof is quite simply a thick piece of skin; part of the epidermal structure, the outermost nonvascular layer that covers and protects the bones within the hoof (Fig. 2-53).

Housed within the hoof are the pedal bone (P3), about half of the short pastern (P2) and the navicular bone (the distal sesamoid). The general name used to identify the entire exterior hoof casing is '*the hoof capsule*' and as the phrase suggests, it surrounds and encapsulates the bones and the accompanying sensitive, highly vascular dermal tissue, which the hoof serves to protect. However the hoof has not only evolved to protect the potentially vulnerable tissue it encloses but also to support the weight of the horse both in stance and throughout its cycle of movement. Its unique but well-defined tasks means it has to be tough, resilient to natural wear and provide a certain amount of flexibility.

The hoof is not usually a regular geometric shape (Fig. 2-54) instead, as a general rule, it is of an asymmetric design and this irregular form must be followed in shoeing. Its principle shape is derived from the pedal bone cocooned within its shell, although it also takes in some form from the soft tissue it surrounds and protects. However, this primal arrangement is subject to change through growth, wear and the influence of force which is imposed upon the hoof by the weight of the horse during stance and movement. It is these factors that collectively create the hoof shape that we see and it this given shape which is commonly known as 'hoof conformation'.

The fact that a range of variables governs the hoof shape and that this shape is then retained, is due to the nature of the horn being predominantly plastic. This idea of the hoof being plastic is something that may not come readily to the reader. However, the term 'plastic' is not just given to objects that are of a synthetic origin, but is also used to define the nature of an object, which has the ability to be moulded or changed in shape. This innate characteristic of the hoof to be moulded by force but also to be then reduced by wear, is the very reason why farriery is essential to the welfare of the equine. The balance of the hoof is not a condition that is static. In an ideal world, the equine hoof would be shaped by stance and reduced by movement, and equilibrium would exist between the two. Unfortunately, the ideal rarely exists and so human intervention, in the form of farriery, is so often needed. Balancing the hoof is frequently considered the main role of the farrier, and his alone, but it is essential to all concerned with the welfare of the horse that we all recognise what the normal hoof is like and know why it is the way it is.

The shape of the hoof wall and hoof capsule when viewed from the front (a craniocaudal view) is now commonly known as mediolateral balance. Ideally, the angle from the top of the hoof to the ground surface should be of a similar angle on both sides (symmetrical) (Fig. 2-55). However, in the normal hoof the angle of the medial side (the side closer to the mid-line of the horse), will be steeper or more upright than the outer-side (lateral side). Looking at the hoof from the side (a lateral view), the anterioposterior balance of the hoof may be assessed (Fig. 2-56). The front of the hoof, the hoof wall, will be considerably longer and higher than the horn at the heel, which will only be about a third of both the length and height of the toe.

The wall is continually growing, migrating down the sensitive tissue within. The wall grows downwards from the coronary band and as it grows downwards and forwards, there is a constant lengthening of the toe. This can effectively bring the bearing surface of the hoof

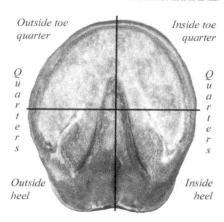

Outside toe quarter   *Inside toe quarter*

Quarters   *Quarters*

Outside heel   *Inside heel*

Fig. 2-54: The palmar view of a right fore hoof, showing an asymmetric but normal form.

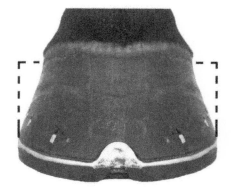

Fig. 2-55: A craniocaudal view of the hoof, showing a symmetrical form.

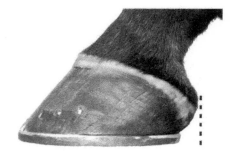

Fig. 2-56: A lateral view of the hoof, with optimal shoe length.

The toe

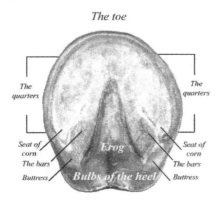

The
quarters

The
quarters

Seat of
corn

The bars

Buttress

Frog

Seat of
corn

The bars

Buttress

Bulbs of the heel

Fig. 2-57: A palmar view of a left fore hoof, identifying some of the named parts.

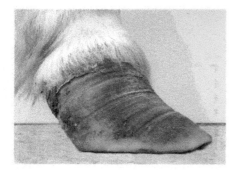

Fig. 2-58: 'Growth rings' or 'laminitic rings'.

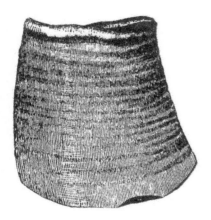

Fig. 2-59: A crooked right fore hoof (taken from Lungwitz, 1884).

out of its proper relationship with the limb, which it supports. Ideally, there should be a balance between growth and wear. Unfortunately, this seldom occurs and it is this continuous interaction which provides the need for farriery. In the shod horse, the hoof wall is not worn away and it continues growing but although the shoe may wear, it may not wear at the same rate as the hoof grows. So again, there is a need for the farrier's attention at regular intervals and with the shod horse that will be about every eight weeks. When the foot is lifted and the hoof is viewed on that plane, it will be seen that the wall of the hoof is thicker at the toe but reduces in thickness as it encompasses the widest part of the hoof (***the quarters***). As it continues towards the heel, it may appear to broaden slightly as it nears the terminal point known as ***the buttress***, where it then returns medially at an angle, to become what is known as ***the bars*** of the hoof. The name given to the area of sole positioned within this angle is known as the seat of corn and this is where areas of bruising can sometimes be seen.

The hoof wall varies only slightly in thickness from its ground surface to its uppermost point of origin and it is this continuous vertical thickness, which allows nails to be driven into the wall to secure a shoe, however its exterior surface is not always smooth.

COMPRESSION MARKS

Although it has been stated that the normal hoof wall remains a constant thickness as it grows down the sensitive tissue and bone which it protects, there are a growing number of authorities, such as the eminent American veterinarian James Rooney DVM, who acknowledge that a slight variation in its thickness occurs due to the wall itself deforming under compression. Compression tends to cause the integrity of the wall to be compromised as it is sandwiched under the weight of the horse and the opposing forces of the ground. Marks can frequently be observed which are often referred to as growth rings or laminitic rings and these are a characteristic trait of compressed deformed horn. These marks or ridges can be seen to run along a plane almost parallel to the coronary border, although frequently these ridges can be seen to converge at the front of the hoof and become wider toward the heel. Although ridges are a familiar sight in the hoof wall, there seems to be little explanation of how or why they occur. A likely and simple explanation can be found when it is understood that the hoof wall is made up of tiny tubules that are bound together. When tube is bent, it has an ingrained prerequisite to become stretched on one side and to buckle on the other, so it is the buckling of the horn tubes, which seems to be the most likely explanation.

Concussion is also considered to play an active role in the deformation of the hoof wall. Bruising to the wall can often be seen in white hooves and the non-pigmented sections of the hoof, particularly in the areas where buckling has occurred and deformation is present. Whatever the cause of deformation, the effects are clearly visible and are evidenced on the hooves of the vast majority of horses and ponies. Illustrations appear in many of the classic texts on horseshoeing depicting this type of deformation but although there has been little attempt to detail explanation about the ridges, it is clear that most farriery authors have considered the major cause to be compression.

THE GROUND SURFACE OF THE HOOF

The sole, frog and the white line are all identifiable and well-known features to those familiar with the horse.

The sole forms the largest part of the hoof, which is exposed to the ground surface and serves to protect the sensitive tissue and bone within. Ideally, it is vaulted or concave and reflects the shape and positioning of the underside of the pedal bone. On a horse where the sole is flatter in form, it is more prone to injury from stones and uneven ground and this can be a major problem. That is why, in certain conditions, it is essential that some horses are shod in order to provide them with protection and comfort: the shoes effectively raising the sole off the ground.

The sole continuously grows from the dermal tissue it protects and as a general rule once it reaches a determined thickness it tends to flake away or exfoliate (Fig. 2-60). However all horses are different and all are exposed to a huge range of variables, some horses have thicker soles than others and in dry environments exfoliation may not readily occur.

The trimming of the sole is something that is both often open to debate and subject to interpretation. However, it is fair to say that during the course of normal farriery it is customary to clean the sole and remove loose tissue prior to making any assessments about trimming.

Bruising to the sole is something that can all too frequently occur, when it does discolouration and actual haemorrhaging may sometimes be seen. Lameness can vary though it is usually in keeping with the obvious extent of the lesion. Corns are another form of bruising but the difference between corns and other types of bruising is that corns are the result of haemorrhaging occurring because of internal damage caused through hoof balance problems (Fig. 2-61).

Corns occur within the angular area between the hoof wall and the bars of the hoof (Fig. 2-62).

Positioned between the medial and lateral bars of the hoof is the triangular mass called the frog, which is made from a tough highly flexible horn. The frog, which is a wedge shaped pad of horn, extends to the rear of the hoof where it forms the part of the hoof known as the bulbs of the heels. Proximally at the transition from skin to horn, its border has a fine covering of a protective layer of horn called periople. The frog is often viewed as a 'barometer' of the hoof indicating its general health and condition. Ideally, it should appear neither overdeveloped (hypertrophied) nor atrophied (underdeveloped), as both extremes are considered problematic and symptomatic of poor hoof balance. In the sound well-balanced hoof, it would seem to maintain a comfortable working height by being raised off the ground by about three eighths of an inch, or 1cm. Its primal shape and form reflects the shape of the corium or sensitive tissue from where it grows.

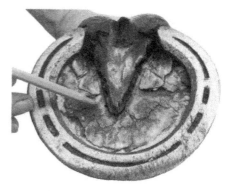

Fig. 2-60: Often it can be seen that when the sole grows to a certain thickness it exfoliates or flakes away (Photo: J. Watts).

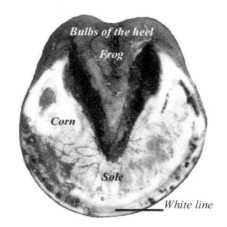

Fig. 2-61: The hoof capsule, showing the site of a 'corn'.

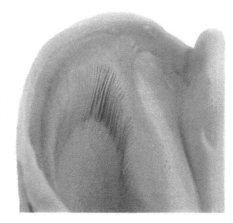

Fig. 2-62: The internal form of the hoof capsule, showing the angular area where haemorrhaging can occur, the result is known as a corn.

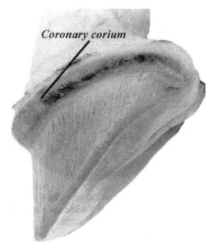

Fig. 2-63: The underlying, germinative, structure of the hoof.

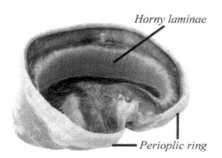

Fig. 2-64: Hoof capsule.

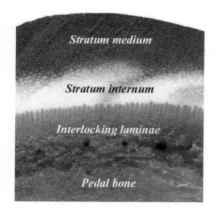

Fig. 2-65: A close-up of a cross-section, showing the dermal and epidermal tissue of the horny wall

The white line is the common term given to the area where the horn of the sole meets the horn of the wall. The white zone, describes an area of non-pigmented horn, which forms part of the connective union between the hoof and the bone and this known as the horny laminae. At the ground surface, the horny laminae connect to and interdigitate with, a yellow horn confusingly called the white line. The white line is an insensitive horn, which is produced by small terminal papillae located at the base of the sensitive laminae, which cover the pedal bone and it is this yellow horn, which provides a flexible junction between sole and wall.

THE PERIOPLIC AND CORONARY CORIUM

The hoof wall grows from the site known as the coronary band and is a continuation of the overlying epidermal layer of skin. The dermis, the principal layer of skin, is rich in blood vessels and life-giving fluids. While the epidermis, the outermost nonvascular layer of skin, starts with layers of active living cells (the germinative layer) these die off, as new cells are formed below to create the hard protective covering of the body.

At the transition of skin and hoof, the dermal papillae become finger-like and all along the coronary corium, thousands of papillae, (cones of cells), droop downwards towards the ground surface, rather like icicles.

In order to ease the transition of pliable skin to ridged hoof, a rubber-like intermediate zone is formed (*the periople*). This soft, light coloured horny layer contains keratohyalin, which is a flexible substance. The perioplic horn, or *Stratum externum*, forms a fine covering which is considered to protect the new horny wall. The main band of this horn is sometimes known as the '*perioplic ring*' and it is located directly above the *coronary corium*. Its distal border is extremely fine and as it nears the ground surface, it has a tendency to become worn away.

The hoof wall structure is formed by the chains of cells, which take their form from the tips of the finger-like papillae covering the coronary corium. These chains of cells form spirally arranged cords, which are known as the horn tubules; these are bound together in a bed of intertubular horn. In this way, the hoof wall is made up of thousands of parallel tubes all held together by a bonding medium, creating that which we know as the hoof wall, the pigmented or non-pigmented *Stratum medium*.

The Stratum medium grows alongside and merges to become fused with the *Stratum internum*, or *Stratum lamellatum*, known commonly in its more familiar term as the *horny laminae*. In dark hooves, on the underside of the hoof, the difference between the two layers of horn is quite distinguishable, as the Stratum internum is without pigment and is much softer. This area is highly susceptible to damage from stones and grit, which can be a major problem and the reason why many horses are shod, simply to protect them from that type of injury.

THE SENSITIVE LAMINAE

The sensitive structures within the hoof are so called because they contain many blood vessels and nerve endings and it is these primary areas that are vulnerable to damage, pain and bleeding.

The sensitive laminae, the dermal laminal corium, cover the anterior surface of the pedal bone (P3). The laminal leaves are arranged in almost parallel vertical rows, are considered to be around six hundred in number, and are known as the primary laminae. Each of the primary laminae is in turn bordered by one to two hundred secondary laminae and as these sensitive laminae interdigitate with the horny laminae they produce a suggested total connective area of approximately one square metre. In fact, it is through this extremely strong union between the bone and the hoof wall that the horse is, in essence, actually suspended up off the ground.

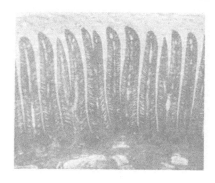

Fig. 2-66: A microscopic view, showing how the dermal and the epidermal laminae interdigitate with one another.

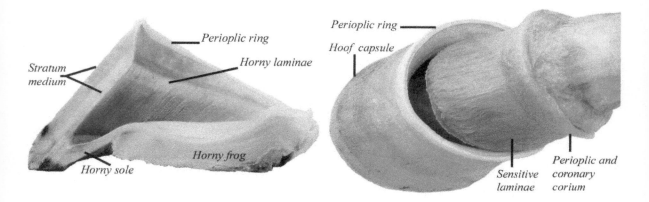

Figs. 2-67: Left, an exposed saggital section of the hoof capsule and right, the dermal tissue exposed.

THE SENSITIVE SOLE

The sensitive sole is the corium or dermal tissue that produces the horny sole. It has a velvety appearance that covers the underside of the pedal bone, which is firmly attached to the bone's periosteal covering.

In much the same way as the coronary band produces the periople and the horny wall, the horny sole is produced by small short papillae, a horn-producing layer of cells called the *Stratum germinativum*.

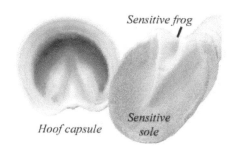

Fig. 2-68: The hoof capsule and the exposed dermal tissue from which it is produced.

THE SENSITIVE FROG

The velvet-like dermal germinative covering which envelops the anterior and the underside or solear surface of the pedal bone extends posteriorly to cover the plantar or digital cushion. Here, once again, short papillae are responsible for producing another specialised type of horn, the horny frog.

In all there are five microscopically different germinative areas that produce subtly different but identifiable specialised types of horn cells. 1: The perioplic ring, producing the periople. 2: The coronary corium, producing the Stratum medium and the Stratum internum. 3: The sensitive laminae, the distal end of the laminal leaves producing the white line. 4: The sensitive sole secreting the horny sole and 5: the sensitive frog, secreting the horny frog.

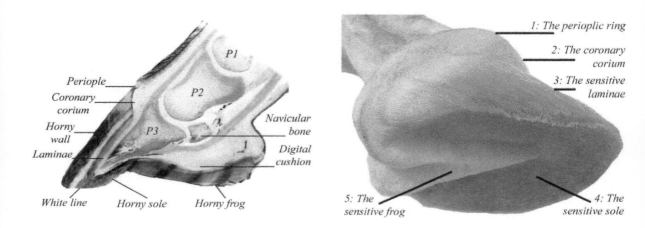

Figs. 2-69: Left, The saggital section of the hoof capsule (Photo supplied by Samuel Beeley, farrier, UK) and right, the germinative areas of the hoof.

THE DIGITAL CUSHION

The digital cushion is a subcutaneous tissue composed of some fatty, connective and fibrous elastic tissue, its wedge shaped form lies beneath the sensitive and horny frog filling the space between the heels of the hoof. Its primal shape is responsible for forming the bulbs of the heels. It is associated with, and adherent to, the deep digital flexor tendon. Distally the medial and lateral borders of the cushion are attached to the collateral cartilages but proximally a venous plexus lies between them.

It is generally accepted that the primary function of the digital cushion is to diminish the effects of concussion.

THE COLLATERAL CARTILAGES

The collateral cartilages, also known as the lateral cartilages, are attached to the medial and lateral wings or palmar processes of the pedal bone (P3). These cartilages, also known as ungual cartilages, are rhomboid shaped plates located on both sides of the hoof with 50% of their form to be found above the coronary band. They are considered to share a variety of functions including being a shield to the underlying structures. They are also considered to play a role in absorbing concussion. They are formed from a mixture of fibrous and hyaline cartilage which has an inherent tendency to become ossified (change to bone); this can either begin through age and repeated trauma or through a sudden injury such as an over-reach, and it is this type of transformation of the cartilages that is commonly known as sidebone.

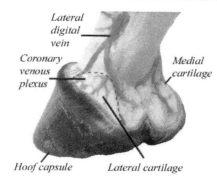

Fig. 2-70: Around 50% of the cartilage can be felt, above the coronary band of the hoof.

THE BARE BONES OF ANATOMY (CONCLUSION)

The real, take-home, message about the anatomy of the horse, its limbs and of course the hoof's structure, is that there is such a lot that both collectively and as individuals, we either don't know or don't understand. We do know however, that being living tissue, it can be damaged and that to repair, if it is repairable, can take quite a long time. Therefore, the best course of action is good management coupled with knowledgeable sympathetic farriery. We know that for every action there is a reaction and that there is always a flip side to every thing we do. We must never ever lose sight of the fact that although we may look at things in isolation and in detail all aspects of the horse should always be viewed as belonging to a single functioning unit. Therefore to help us remember this single salient point we need only think about the haunting African/American spiritual song we probably all learnt at school and recall the words of Ezekiel because everything is connected.

Your toe bone's connected to your foot bone.
Your foot bone's connected to your anklebone.
Your anklebone's connected to your leg bone.
Your leg bone's connected to your thighbone.
Your thighbone's connected to your hipbone.
Your hipbone's connected to your backbone.
Your backbone's connected to your shoulder bone.
Your shoulder bone's connected to your neck bone.
Your neck bone's connected to your head bone.

So, just think...remember...everything is connected!

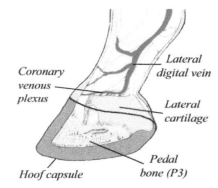

Fig. 2-71: Illustration showing the positioning of the cartilage within the hoof capsule.

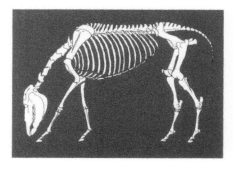

Fig. 2-72: The bare bones of farriery. Farriery needs to consider everything!

BIBLIOGRAPHY

'If you take ideas from one source it's called plagiarism. When you take ideas from five it's called research'

Adams, O.R., *Lameness in Horses* (Lea & Febiger; Philadelphia, 1979)

Axe, J.W., *The Horse, its treatment in Health and Disease* (Gresham Publishing Company Co. London, 1905)

Back, W., Clayton, H. M., *Equine Locomotion* (Harcourt Publishers Ltd 2001)

Bennett, D., *Principles of Equine Orthopedics: Stance and Biomechanics for Every Horse* Owner (The Inner Horseman; newsletter of Equine Studies Institute © 2001-2003 by Deb Bennett, Ph.D.)

Blood, D.C., Studdart, V.P., *Baillière's Comprehensive Veterinary Dictionary* (Baillière Tindall, 1988)

Clayton, H.M., *'Practical aspects of the equine gait analysis'* (The Fourth International Farriery and Lameness seminar 1994 Handbook, p.9-11)

Clayton, H.M., *The Science of Lameness* (Veterinary Connection: USDF Connection, September 2001, p.29-32)

Codrington, W.S., *Know Your Horse: a guide to selection and care in health and disease* (J.A. Allen & Co. London S.W.1; revised edition 1966)

Duhousset, E., *The Gaits, Exterior and Proportions of the Horse* (Percy Young, Gower Street, 1896)

Dyson, S.J., *Pain Associated with the Sacroiliac Joint Region: A Diagnostic Challenge* (50th Annual Convention of the American Association of Equine Practitioners, 2004, Denver Colorado)

Ellenberger, W., Dittrich, H., Baum, H., *An Atlas of Animal Anatomy for Artists* (Dover Publications, Inc., New York, 2nd edition 1956)

Emery, L., Miller, J., Van Hoosen, N., *Horseshoeing Theory and Hoof Care* (Lea & Febiger, 1977)

Freeman, S., *Observations on the Mechanism of the Horse's Foot*, 1796.

Goody, P.C., *'Horse Anatomy; a pictorial approach to equine structure'* (J. A. Allen London 1983)

Gray, H., *Gray's Anatomy* (Bounty Books: New York, 1977)

Green, J., *Horse Anatomy* (Dover Publications, Inc., Mineola, New York, 2006)

Green, J., *Horses, CD-ROM & BOOK* (Dover Publications, Inc., Mineola, New York, 2003)

Harris, S.H., *Horse Gaits Balance and Movement* (Macmillan Publishing Co. 1993)

Hayes, M.H., *Points of the Horse* (Arco Publishing Company, Inc., 1976)

Hickman, J., Humphrey, M., *Hickman's Farriery* (J.A. Allen & Co. Ltd, 1988)

Kainer, R.A., McCracken, T.O., *Horse Anatomy, a Coloring Atlas* (Alpine Publications, Loveland, Colorado; 2nd edition 1998)

Keegan, K.G., *Pelvic Movement Pattern in Horses with Hindlimb and Forelimb Lameness* (In-Depth: Lameness in Motion: AAEP Proceedings/ Vol.51/2005)

Lawrence, R., *An inquiry into the Structure and Animal Economy of the Horse* (Robert Baldwin, Paternoster Row, London 1803)

Ridgway, K.J., *'Low Heel/High Heel Syndrome Effects on the Shoulder'* (A BRIDGE TO THE FUTURE Veterinary Conference, August, 2003, August 10, 2003)

Rooney, J.R., *THE LAME HORSE; Causes, Symptoms, and Treatment* (Melvin Powers, Wilshire Book Company, 1974)

Smythe, R.H., Goody, P.C., *Horse Structure and Movement* (J. A. Allen, London, 2nd edition 1975)

Smythe, R.H., Goody, P.C., *Horse Structure and Movement* (J.A. Allen, London, 3rd edition, revised by Peter Gray MVB MRCVS, 1993)

Stashak, T.S., *Adams' Lameness in Horses* (Lea & Febiger, 4th edition 1987)

Stewart Hastie, P., *The BHS Veterinary Manual* (Kenilworth Press 2001)

Thacker, P., *'Trimming to Achieve Pastern Axis Alignment vs. Trimming to Match Angle Pairs'* (Contradictions in Current Horseshoeing Theory) http://www.hopeforsoundness.com/miscfiles/Thacker-Mismatchedfeet.pdf (Access March, 2007)

Thompson, E. E., *Anatomy of Animals; studies in the forms of mammals and birds* (Bracken Books, London 1996)

3: Hoof balance revealed

BIOMECHANICS IN FARRIERY

In the daily scheme of things, the farrier would seem to have many roles. Certainly, the principal role of the farrier is to put shoes on horses to stop their feet from wearing out and when the farrier's role is viewed in those terms, his tasks are clearly undervalued. There is definitely more to farriery than simply putting shoes on. Farriers have to have some idea of what response their efforts may make to the hooves that they work upon. Owners also need to be aware of what results may be expected both for when things go right and for when things go wrong. Vets need to know that the shoes or treatment they recommend will provide the results they want for their clients.

The role of the farrier should be a benign one, causing minimal damage to the hooves when applying shoes and a positive role trimming the horn of the hooves that are overgrown or out of balance. New technology arrives daily and most farriers are constantly refining their skills and acquiring new ones. Biomechanics, kinematics and kinetics are all relatively new phrases and sciences, which are rapidly being recognised as being essential to understand fully the role of farriery.

Equine biomechanics is a science that applies the use of mechanical laws and principles to explain and understand the horse's movements and the results of those movements during equine locomotion. Kinematics and kinetics are two interrelated but separately defined studies, which come under the umbrella of equine biomechanics. Kinematics looks at the ranges of movement in both time and space while kinetics looks at the forces involved. Biomechanical analysis is available in laboratories and research centres which use technical equipment and sophisticated computer software. Currently these places are limited and for most are both prohibitively expensive and unnecessary.

Understanding not only how the hoof is structurally formed but also how that structure can be deformed is a phenomenon of which we all as guardians of the horse should have some perception. Independently, we can all make the effort to build up a better understanding even without hi-tech equipment simply through observation and reason; this is essential.

It may seem obvious, but the main object of farriery is to make the horse as comfortable as possible when the hooves are on the ground bearing the weight of the horse plus any load it may be given at times to carry. Here in the UK the majority of horses are ridden, so farriery has to account for both horse and rider and the terrain over which the animal is expected to travel. To begin to appreciate the forces placed upon the limb we need to look at and analyse the biomechanics of stance, both during the act of progression and at rest.

PROGRESSION

The gaits of the horse are isolated, descriptively defined and identified phases of movement, designed to help us understand the movements of progression. A gait is a cyclical pattern of movement recognised by the sequence and timing of footfalls, one complete cycle of hoof and limb movement forming the action known as a 'stride'.

During each stride there is a period when the hoof is in contact with the ground, this is known as the stance phase (Fig.3-1). The stance phase begins as the hoof strikes the ground. As each animal has its own distinctive pattern of movement and the environmental conditions are subject to a whole range of variables, it has to be expected that the hooves of any animal may make contact with the ground with one aspect of the hoof or another. It has been assumed that the ideal hoof should land flat, however, it is generally accepted that horses that display a normal hoof conformation, and those which exhibit more upright hooves may both land heel first. Flat hooves may land toe first although this type of footfall tends to be associated with lameness. Unfortunately, there is no definitive law about which aspect of the hoof should land first. The way the hoof is trimmed (hoof balance) is considered to play a major role and so too is the gait in which the animal is moving and at what speed. Another considered opinion is that proprioceptive reflexes have a role in determining footfall. Proprioceptory nerve endings provide essential information about movements and positioning of the body and so it is thought the hoof may land according to the position of the pedal bone rather than the surrounding hoof capsule (Figs. 3-2).

After the initial contacts, the hoof and limb enter the stance phase proper. At the time of initial impact, the limb could be described as being fully extended, although as the limb prepares for the hoof to make contact with the ground it enters a state of deceleration and retraction in order to minimise the concussive effects of impact. As the initial contact with the ground surface takes place, there is a period between impact and coming to rest which is known as the 'slide time' or 'slip distance', and is part of the deceleration process. When the hoof becomes stationary relative to the ground, it enters an expected and recognised pattern of movement as the body of the horse moves forward over the limb. Once the hoof is in a stationary position, the limb continues to decelerate, dissipating the forward force of momentum through the dynamic structure of the hoof and through the extension of the fetlock as the joint sinks towards the ground. As the pastern descends closer to the ground, energy is stored within the flexor tendons and suspensory ligament that will later be released during the period of acceleration in the second half of the stance phase, after the limb has been maximally loaded. During the maximal

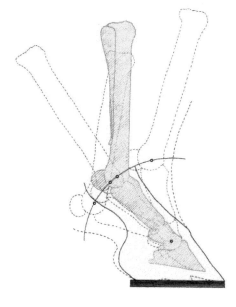

Fig. 3-1: The Stance Phase

The stance phase is the term given to the period when the hoof is placed flat to the ground, supporting the animal's bodyweight, during the act of progression.

There are two distinct phases, the first phase is the period between impact and mid-stance; this is a period of deceleration; absorbing concussion and storing energy. The second phase is one of acceleration, when stored energy is released from tendons and ligaments; this action occurs between mid-stance and heel-off.

extension of the fetlock and throughout the entire stance phase, the main body of the horse passes over the static hoof, with the limb acting as a series of levers and the pedal joint serving as the principal fulcrum throughout this action (Fig. 3-3).

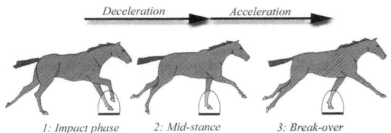

1: Impact phase   *2: Mid-stance*   *3: Break-over*

Fig. 3-3: The Stance Phase

As the hoof of the equine strikes the ground during the act of progression, it assumes the attitude described as the impact phase (1) and this phase is one of deceleration. Once the pastern has descended maximally and the cannon bone is vertical to the ground surface, then the limb assumes the mid-stance position (2). From this point the limb enters the period of acceleration, during this period and when the limb achieves the limits allowed by the fetlock, pastern and pedal joints it enters the phase known as 'breakover' and this phase starts as the stance phase ends, at heel-off (3).

SIMPLE MECHANICS: THE ORIGINS OF BIOMECHANICS

A fulcrum is a fixed point around which a lever turns and it serves us well to remember that during the stance phase, the entire body of the horse will pivot around this joint. In the first half of the stance phase, the combined structure formed by the long and the short pastern creates a lever arm and the action created is that of a third class lever.

Levers form an integral part of our daily lives, they are around us everywhere and can be found in the things we use each and every day; door handles, scissors, the pedals in our cars, all of these are formed by levers.

The laws of simple mechanics may seem far removed from farriery and veterinary practices but to understand the functional anatomy of the equine, the horse must be viewed as a complex machine. However, just like all other complex machines the mechanics involved can be isolated and broken down into simple actions and components. This type of reasoning is far from new.

Leonardo da Vinci (1452-1519) artist and inventor had a deep interest in the movements of animals. As an anatomist, he studied and dissected many cadavers and then painstakingly drew them and throughout these studies, he is known to have described the body as a machine. He also went to great lengths to illustrate how joints worked by replacing muscles with strings so that he could demonstrate how,

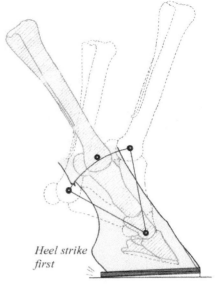

Heel strike first

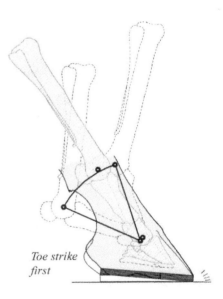

Toe strike first

Figs. 3-2: Illustration depicting the impact phase of the upright and flat hooves

As the hoof strikes the ground at the start of the stance phase, it may do so with any aspect. However, it is generally accepted that normal or upright hooves may land heel first, whilst flat hooves may land toe first. It is thought this may be due to the positioning of the pedal bone rather than the surrounding hoof capsule.

First-class lever

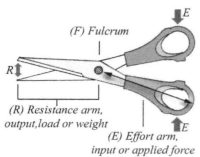

(F) Fulcrum

*(R) Resistance arm,
output, load or weight*

*(E) Effort arm,
input or applied force*

Fig. 3-4a.

Second-class lever

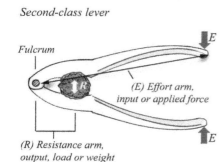

Fulcrum

*(E) Effort arm,
input or applied force*

*(R) Resistance arm,
output, load or weight*

Fig. 3-4b.

Third-class lever

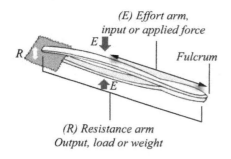

*(E) Effort arm,
input or applied force*

Fulcrum

*(R) Resistance arm
Output, load or weight*

Fig. 3-4c.

combined with the levers formed by bones, they worked to produce motion. Others continued with similar lines of research and study but it was Giovanni Alphonso Borelli (1608-1679), a professor of mathematics at Pisa University, who was to publish his book *De Motu Animalium (On the Movement of Animals, 1681).* This book, considered by many to be ahead of its time, was the first major contribution to the science of equine locomotion since Aristotle (384-322 BC). The importance of leverage has been recognised and understood by anatomists for centuries; its relevance is something that must never be overlooked because the law of levers is without doubt, the backbone of all biomechanics.

LEVERS

The idea shared by scientists and anatomists over the centuries that joints are made up of levers and fulcrums is a concept that has largely failed to be thoroughly explored in the farriery and veterinary world and this is possibly because of its seemingly obvious and simplistic nature. However, just as Borelli recognised that the body can be likened to a machine with the limbs acting as levers, so too have other authors fostered the same conception. In fact, since Borelli the analogy of the limbs being likened to a system of levers has gained popularity. Despite this accepted recognition however, the principals involved have generally been confined within the abstract of levers and fulcrums being simply a part of the mechanism used to provide propulsion. It would seem few authors have clearly attempted to examine and define how those forces created by the levers within the limb can have a determining influence, which will effectively change the shape of the equine hoof. In fact, more often when its application is viewed within the realms of farriery, the principal of levers and fulcrums is used in techniques that are thought to 'correct' limb conformation but it is rarely considered that the conformation of the limb in turn, will affect hoof shape.

A lever is a rigid bar that rotates around a fixed point, which is known as a fulcrum (F). Force is applied at some point and this applied energy is often referred to as effort (E). As a result, the bar exerts force to move a weight or overcome a resistance (R). The distance between the point of effort and the fulcrum (E-F) is called the effort or input arm and the distance between the fulcrum and the resistance is called the resistance or output arm (F-R). What any lever is capable of will depend upon where along the bar the effort, fulcrum and resistance are situated. Levers fall into three distinct types and these can be categorised by their function. In the first-class lever, the fulcrum is set between the effort and the resistance; examples include a crowbar, balance scales and a pair of scissors (Fig. 3-4a). In both the second-class and third-class levers, the effort and the resistance are on the same side of the fulcrum. In the second-class lever, the resistance is between the fulcrum and the effort, as in a pair of nutcrackers (Fig. 3-4b). In the third class lever, the effort is between the fulcrum and the resistance as in the use of a pair of tweezers (Fig. 3-4c).

CLEARER PERCEPTIONS

The mechanics involved within farriery initially appear straightforward and easy to understand but as further study evolves the subject as a whole can be quite overwhelming. Researchers and academics often present to the student a complex and mathematical approach. However, much is not known or fully understood and there is frequent controversy and speculation even amongst those who study this particular field of enquiry. A non-mathematical view of the subject matter is therefore needed both to provide explanations that are of a more tangible nature and to develop a clearer perception of the mechanics involved because a better understanding will then have wide implications upon the future use of farriery as a manipulative procedure.

IMPACT TO MID-STANCE

Throughout the stance phase, the hoof exerts a force against the ground, and in response to this action, the ground exerts a force against the hoof (Newton's third law: 'For every action there is an equal and opposite reaction'). For descriptive and identification purposes this action is often referred to as the 'ground reaction force' (GRF), which is a force that is made up of two principal components, magnitude and direction. Simplified this can be described as the weight of the horse acting upon the limb to produce a vertical component and the actions of deceleration and acceleration producing a horizontal component. Researchers with sophisticated equipment are able to measure both these elements and then use the information to create graphs or diagrams that illustrate both the direction and magnitude of the force relative to the limb's skeletal structure.

At impact, the centre of pressure (COP) is focused upon the initial point of contact at the heels. As the horse travels over the hoof it rises quickly and smoothly toward the centre of the ground surface of the foot, where it remains until approximately 75% of the weight-bearing phase has passed, after which it travels forwards toward the toe and breakover. This action, when measured, can be plotted creating a force-time curve, which ends up looking like an upturned U. The magnitude of the vertical component is low at the initial contact and at breakover but is comparatively higher as it peaks during the middle of the stance. The horizontal component however is considerably smaller with a negative phase (the braking element) and a positive phase (the propulsive element). In addition to these aspects of the ground reaction force, high-frequency vibrations occur during the initial impact phase, which take some 50 milliseconds to disappear and it is these vibrations, which are considered the greatest cause of injury to the athletic horse. Therefore, it is essential that this potential source of physical damage is positively managed by applying well-considered farriery strategies designed to minimise these effects.

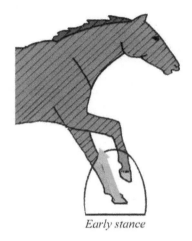

Early stance

Figs. 3-5: Force vectors (arrows), representing a snapshot of both the magnitude and direction of the opposing ground reaction force (GRF), in early and mid-stance.

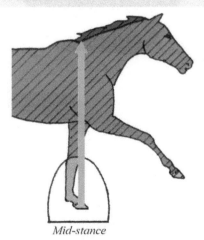

Mid-stance

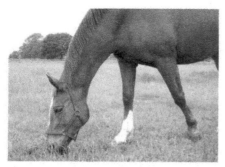

Fig. 3-6: Habits of stance affect hoof shape.

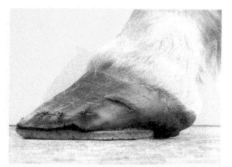

Fig. 3-7: A flat or collapsed hoof.

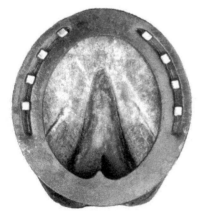

Fig. 3-8: An egg-bar shoe.

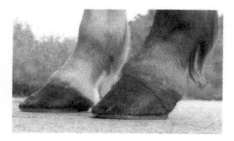

Fig. 3-9: A pair of hooves exhibiting strikingly dissimilar hoof shapes.

FARRIERY AND THE CAUDAL HOOF

The hoof is a semi-rigid structure with a shape that is predominantly influenced by the weight of the horse during the act of stance while the horse is at rest. Its shape, being conformed by one pattern of action (stance at rest), then has to accommodate other patterns of action, impact, mid-stance and breakover (during progression). Progression is initiated through the sequences of a range of structured movements and it is through these actions, that other modifications then take place.

The patterns of stance at rest (Fig. 3-6) and the effects those patterns have over hoof shape is a subject which has sadly received scant attention, unlike the study of motion which has been studied in depth. This has mainly been because an understanding of locomotion is commonly accepted to be the only necessary knowledge essential in leading to a better appreciation of the mechanics of lameness. This has in turn influenced the way many of those studies have looked at the role which farriery has had to play in alleviating those lamenesses.

In the UK, long toes and low heels (Fig. 3-7) are considered a major problem regarding hoof balance, having a deep association with lameness. Historically this has prompted attention to be aimed at reducing the toe length with a view to easing breakover and raising the heels in an effort to relieve excessive strain on the deep digital flexor tendon. However, recent areas of research have highlighted that some of the most seemingly beneficial practices have not consistently proved as successful as commonly reported. This may be because some practices focus on corrective measures rather than preventative management.

Caudal hoof pain including navicular disease, ligament damage and tendon injuries are conditions that are traditionally managed through set farriery practices. These practices principally involve either raising the heels or extending the shoe's length and sometimes a combination of both is applied.

Raising the heels has been shown to unload the deep digital flexor tendon reducing the force applied to navicular bone. However, by raising the heels, the force upon the heels is increased and the base of support provided by the shoe is frequently compromised.

Egg-bar shoes are sometimes recommended as an alternative (Fig. 3-8); these extend the base of support and have been effective in helping those hooves that are considered flat or have been identified as having collapsed heels. Although the mechanism of the action has not been fully explained it has been assumed that by extending the base of support, the hoof is able to redistribute its load over a larger area, which then makes full use of the heel's structure and the reinforcement/coupling of the flexible caudal regions of the foot.

Intriguingly, low/weak-heeled hooves and strong/upright hooves (Fig. 3-9) have both been linked to navicular disease and caudal heel pain. Early researchers suggested narrow/boxy hooves were the cause of these disorders but later modern researchers considered that flat hooves were the important predisposing factor. This shift in opinion grew and prompted the explanation that some horses with long standing navicular disease went on to develop boxy, upright feet.

Adjusting the caudal length of a shoe has been proven to be effective in influencing the forces imposed upon the heels. It is this evidence, which helps support the reasoning that the caudal aspects of the hoof act in association to assist as contributing agents in providing the effort needed to support the horse off the ground as the fetlock descends. This identifying action, of the weight of the horse acting as a load, the caudal regions responding as an effort and the pedal joint acting as a fulcrum, establishes the joint a third-class lever (Fig. 3-10).

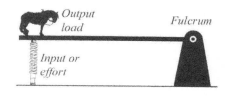

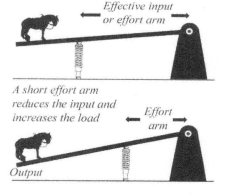

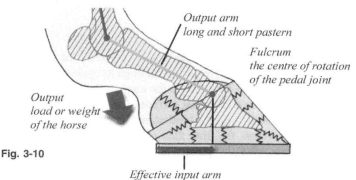

Fig. 3-10

As a third-class lever the effort is supplied by the combined effects of bone, tendon, horn, sole, frog, digital cushion, cartilage and numerous ligaments.

Fig. 3-11: A third-class lever. The most caudal aspect of the shoe or, where a shoe is not applied, the hoof, defines the length of the effective effort arm.

A short shoe multiplies the effective load and reduces the effective effort available to support it. While too long a shoe would, in theory, convert the action to that of a second-class lever, which would then directly apply a force that could also crush the heels.

Operating as a third-class lever the caudal aspect of the shoe will have an optimal length. Too long a shoe will convert the lever's action and apply pressure to the heels, while too short a shoe will cause the fetlock to hyper-extend and induce an increased flexion of the pedal joint.

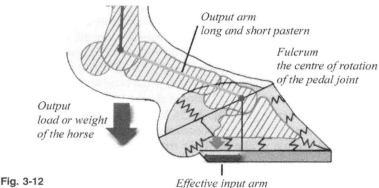

Fig. 3-12

Effective input arm

Applying too short a shoe to weak/flat hooves will produce obvious effects, as a short shoe will increase the effect of the horse's weight and cause the heels to collapse; this is caused by a plastic deformation, due to the viscoelastic nature of the hoofs structure (Fig. 3-12). On the other hand, structurally strong hooves may not deform under the load and the effects can go unnoticed until the horse becomes lame.

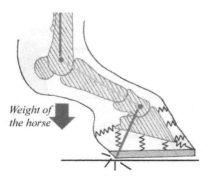

Fig. 3-13: Too short a heel can become a pivotal point during stance.

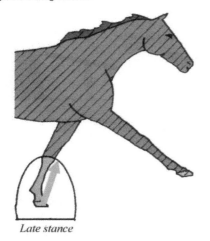

Fig. 3-14: A snapshot of the GRF during late stance (second half of the stance phase).

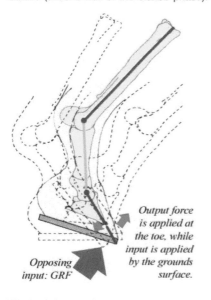

Fig. 3-15: The actions of breakover.

Upon impact, strong upright-heeled hooves are more likely to be affected by concussive forces as they contact the ground; however, their boxy shape may also create another effect, which should provide another area of concern. This is because their ground-surface contact area can be effectively too far forward which creates a pivotal effect that could, in theory, lead to a hyperextension of the fetlock joint and an increased flexion of the pedal joint (Fig. 3-13). Although speculative, could this inherent instability provide the link that unites both upright/strong hooves and flat/weak hooves to be associated with caudal hoof pain and navicular disease?

MID-STANCE TO BREAKOVER

Once the fetlock has descended maximally, it reaches the theoretical point of zero motion (PZM). This occurs through its cycle of movement and is considered to take place when the cannon bone has reached a vertical position (90° to the ground surface); the limb is then deemed to have reached what is called the 'mid-stance' position. After adopting the mid-stance position, the limb then enters the second half of the stance phase, releasing the energy stored within the tendons and ligaments (Fig. 3-14).

During the moments that the heels prepare to leave the ground, the distal limb takes on the form of a first-class lever. This occurs because the pedal joint's centre of rotation repeats its role as a fulcrum and the toe of the hoof takes on the form of a resistance arm (output) while the effort (input) is derived from the horse's body weight; this results in an output force being applied at the toe. The result of this action is for the hoof to be pushed in a downward and backwards motion while the ground applies an opposite input force against the hoof wall.

As breakover begins, priorities and emphases change, both because of the action and because of the structural elements that make up this semi-rigid lever. The instant the heels leave the ground, the toe of the hoof becomes a fulcrum, with the effort still coming from the forward momentum of the horse; the load (output) is applied to the semi-rigid lever of the toe. This action pushes the pedal bone in a downward and backwards rotation, while the horn at the toe is opposed by the input from the grounds surface (Fig. 3-15). It is this action, which gives the hoof its final push off and it is because of this action that the demands upon this section of the hoof are truly put to the test. As the toe becomes a pivotal point, a frictional force takes place creating the abrading wear pattern frequently described as breakover. In barefoot horses, growth ideally replaces this wear or in shod horses, the shoe prevents it. However, where the growth is too long or there is disunity with this semi-rigid lever, horn breakage or deformity can occur.

FARRIERY AND BREAKOVER

Breakover is the descriptive phrase given to the period of movement that takes place as first the heel and then the toe of the hoof leaves contact with the ground. 'Heel-off' occurs as the fetlock, pastern and pedal joints reach their extreme range of movement in the final part of the stance phase. As the body of the horse is projected forward, the heel of the hoof is forced to rise off the ground, pushing the toe of the hoof into the ground surface.

To reduce or ease the breakover is considered by many to be good practice and the logic would seem to be obvious; however there are conflicting opinions about the application of this idea. This may be explained by saying that all hooves are different and that all farriers have different work practices, nevertheless the benefits remain sketchy and unproven.

The term 'breakover' defines not only the action but also the effects, with the main affect being the wear pattern at the toe.

As suggested, as the action takes place, wear occurs to the toe, which has prompted some authorities to suggest that if the hoof wears in such a way then that is the way it should be shod. However, during test conditions, both on a hard surface and on a rubber floor, horses shod with rocker, rolled and square-toed shoes (simulating theoretical wear patterns), did not achieve any significantly different breakover duration times, when compared to those shod in a more normal and traditional manner. It has even been considered that actively attempting to encourage or ease breakover by the fitting of such shoes may even produce a negative effect, particularly if the shoeing plan does not reflect the individuals unique wear pattern. This is because attempts at influencing breakover can, it has been suggested, create torsional forces both before and after toe-off causing the hoof to deform and to deviate from its desired swing pattern.

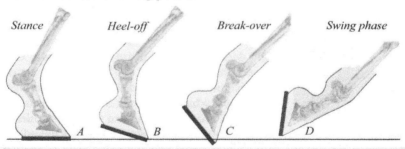

Stance   *Heel-off*   *Break-over*   *Swing phase*

The breakover phase occurs during the moments between the stance phase (when the hoof is flat on the ground), and the swing phase (when the hoof is travelling through the air). It begins as the stance phase ends (**A**). The heel of the hoof is simply levered off the ground as the body of the horse travels forward and the fetlock, pastern and pedal joints reach the limits of their forward range of movement; at this point the action is known as heel-off (**B**).

The act of breakover (**C**) occurs with extreme rapidity too fast for the human eye to perceive, lifting the limb and allowing the knee to flex and move forward. At lift-off (also known as toe off), the tendons and ligaments rebound releasing a final burst of energy, resulting in something like a catapult reaction. This recoil action provides the animal with a final 'push-off' which terminates as the toe of the hoof is flicked back and becomes airborne. With the hoof off the ground, the limb now enters the swing phase (**D**).

CONFORMATION

Horses are often viewed as objects with a leg at each corner but as anyone will tell you, if you were to remove one leg from a table, it would fall over. The maintenance of both the equilibrium and balance of the horse is now considered to be one of the roles associated with farriery today. However, just as suggesting that farriery is simply about putting shoes on is both an understatement and a misinterpretation, then it is also as equally misleading to suggest that farriery has the power alone to correct a whole variety of inherent tendencies and conditions. Horses are individuals with their own unique patterns of movement and behaviour and the most obvious of these identifiable differences can be viewed when looking at the horse either from the front or from behind. Conformation is the term given to a horse's general appearance. When conformation is assessed, a great deal of information is observed and considered. Conformation is judged by size and symmetry, the shape and relative proportions of the various body regions, the straightness of limbs and the flight patterns those limbs create. Conformation is about the appearance of an animal and the observer's appreciation of what he or she considers desirable. Those desirable qualities may make a huge difference both to the performance and to the value of any animal. The saying 'you can't make a silk purse out a sows ear' is very true but a more relevant truth is closer to home 'you can't make a horse better than its best' and owners, farriers and veterinarians should never lose sight of this. Shoeing styles and objectives should always consider the animal's individual conformation and how best to introduce or maintain harmony within the physical makeup of each and every individual horse. There are laws and rules, which are given, but the main one in farriery is not to impose force.

Often when judging an animal's conformation or assessing soundness, the horse will be viewed both coming towards and moving away from the observer. This type of inspection is carried out with the horse either at walk or at trot (Fig. 3-17). The procedure allows the observer to analyse uneven weight bearing and the straightness of flight during the swing phase of locomotion. Equal weight bearing between the limbs is ideal and when it does not occur, to the trained eye it is quite readily spotted because of the uneven shifting of the bodyweight, which will occur. Straight patterns of movement created by the hoof and limb are also considered ideal and a sign that a particular animal is less likely to be predisposed to joint wear and tear than another which may not move quite as straight. However not all animals will, or can, move straight and not all animals will, or can, distribute weight on each limb in the same way as its corresponding partner can.

Conformation is, as the name suggests, the result of the act of conformity. The horse will develop from a foal through to maturity by a process of both nature and nurture. By the time the foal is born, its development has already begun. Joint surfaces and the relative positions they assume have already been decided, so the direction each joint is facing has already been fixed, or 'cast in stone'. From the

Fig. 3-17: Viewing the horse moving to and away from the observer can, to the trained eye, provide a lot of detailed information. (Photograph courtesy J. Watts)

moment the foal stands the limbs will be subject to that inescapable force, gravity. There are thought to be many influences involved in the development of the horse but gravity and inherent characteristics (genetics) are without doubt the main two. Therefore, with the direction of each joint being predetermined and the foal's habits of behaviour being genetically inherent, we need to consider how these two elements combine to create the animal's conformation.

GRAVITY AND EQULIBRIUM

Gravity is a force, which is a constant, being both active and evident in stance and movement. Equilibrium is the phrase given to the management of force and this is achieved as the horse manipulates its body throughout both locomotion and stance. The horse succeeds in this accomplishment by the shifting of its bodyweight and the continued repositioning of its base of support. In doing so, it actively maintains both posture and balance (Fig. 3-18).

The horse is a quadruped but that does not mean that it consistently has four evenly spaced limbs. Throughout its normal phases of movement, it needs to constantly manage a base of support to maintain its bodily position and it does this without any real conscious thought.

Handedness or sidedness and its effects is a subject which has seldom been considered by veterinarians or farriers alike but most horse owners are aware of their horse having a preferred way of going. Not all owners however are aware that their horse may have a preferred way of standing or grazing. Horses with differing sized hooves may have lameness problems but they may also exhibit differing sized hooves simply because they have a dominant side and it is this phenomenon, which may be referred to as the animal being one-sided or 'handed'. Their hooves become different in size and shape because the hoof is compliant to force and the hoof is under constant force whilst it bears weight. However in the foal, there is also another plastic tissue, which is influenced by force and that is the epiphyseal cartilage or growth plate.

The epiphyseal plate is a thin layer of cartilage between the epiphysis and the shaft of a long bone (Fig.3-19). It is an area of growth responsible for the lengthening of the bone, which through age becomes hardened and fused to the main body of bone (epiphyseal closure). As soon as the foal stands, the weight of the animal can and does, have an influential effect upon the formation of new bone and it is this action, which is one of the deciding factors of both conformation and movement. So when the horse is viewed walking to or from the observer what can be seen both in the placement of the hooves and in the swing phase or flight pattern of the hooves is, in the sound horse, the result of its conformation. Therefore, any seemingly undesirable signature of movement may, in fact, simply be a fingerprint or reflection of an individual conformation and to attempt to alter these natural movements through shoeing may not prove to be positive or provide a desirable effect.

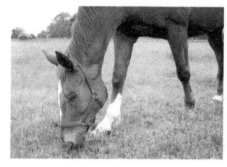

Fig. 3-18: Throughout stance and movement, hooves and limbs are positioned to support the horse's bodyweight.

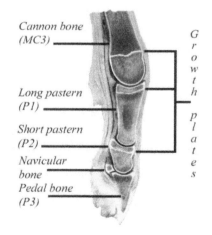

Cannon bone (MC3)

Long pastern (P1)

Short pastern (P2)

Navicular bone

Pedal bone (P3)

G r o w t h p l a t e s

Fig. 3-19: Photograph showing a saggital section of a foal's lower limb, identifying the locations of the epiphyseal plates. Some reports suggest that the closure of these plates can occur as early as 6 months.

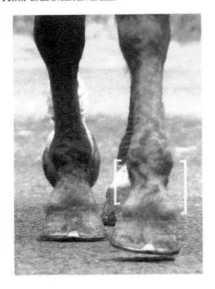

Fig. 3-20: Lateral footfall may be considered undesirable. However, for the individual it may be considered quite normal, influenced both by joint dynamics and hoof shape.

In the picture above it can be seen that in this snapshot, with the distal joints preparing to impact the ground, the medial side of the pastern length would appear to be shorter than the lateral side.

(Photograph courtesy J. Watts)

FOOTFALL

Mediolateral balance has until the last decade or so been an aspect of hoof care and limb balance which has received marginal attention. Experts are currently divided into two camps. There are those that consider the hoof should be trimmed and shod to the long axis of the cannon bone and those who think that trimming and shoeing should be determined by how the hooves contact the ground. The latter type of assessment is sometimes referred to as dynamic balancing. Both schools of thought are very similar as both suggest that when the farrier comes to trim the hooves of any horse he will probably need to trim more off the lateral side than the medial and this may be a requirement if the hoof is to land flat. Assessing footfall is speculative at best, flat footfall may be considered desirable but one thing is clear, hooves that contact lateral heel first may actually be quite normal (Fig.3-20).

The whole progress of footfall is the same whether viewed from the side or from the front; impact is part of the deceleration process and only moments occur between the initial impact and the stance phase proper. When viewed from the side the fetlock can be observed as it descends to become maximally loaded and this action is part of a series of labour saving actions created to absorb force and store energy. These sequential phases of movements are designed to provide an economy of effort and maintain the equine's centre of gravity throughout locomotion, in a relatively unchanged parallel location above the ground. To do this, the distal joints and the fetlock in particular, not only have to move backwards and forwards but also have to accommodate lateral movement as well, and this is provided by their three-dimensional design

DISTAL JOINT MECHANICS

The fetlock is a ginglymus joint, or hinge joint (Fig. 3-21). Many view this joint as having motion in only one plane and that is how the author of the classic text on human anatomy describes this type of joint. However, within the text of *Grays Anatomy* the author states, *'the direction which the distal bone takes in this motion is never in the same plane as that of the axis of the proximal bone, but there is always a certain amount of alteration from the straight line during flexion'*. In effect, this means that the relationship between the axes of each bone is constantly under change as movement occurs.

The fetlock joint has its form dominated by a narrow surface known as the median ridge. This central ridge is located between two other much broader surfaces, known as the medial and lateral condyles. These two condyles are irregular in shape, with the medial condyle being the larger of the two (Fig. 3-22), while the lateral condyle presents a slightly smaller articular surface. Positioned either side of the median ridge, the condyles are eccentrically attached to the central shaft, providing the joint with an articular surface designed not only to accommodate a range of dorsal and palmar movements but to simultaneously perform a subtle range of medial and lateral movements. This amazing, complex joint, seemingly rigid in its design, permits controlled three-dimensional motion. The joint's rigidity provides the strength to support the equine throughout its forward/backward motion and its cam design allows the supporting hoof or hooves to be positioned in such a way that a central base of support is maintained throughout all of the equine gaits.

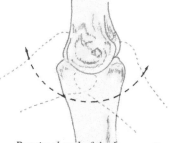

Distal end of the cannon bone

Proximal end of the long pastern

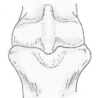

Cannon (MC3)

Long pastern (P1)

*The fetlock joint is often considered to have motion in only one plane; forwards and backwards but that description belies it's full range of motion.

Fig. 3-21: lillustrations depicting the basic range of motion of the fetlock joint. (After, Emery, Miller and Van Hoosen, 1977).

The fetlock is a ginglymus, or hinge joint, which is considered by many as having motion in only one plane. However, in the normal limb, the range of motion is a little more dynamic. It is likely that through its subtle but complex design it follows a motion, which allows the hoof to be positioned close to the midline of progression during the stance phase but then during breakover assists in the hoof being directed away from the midlin.

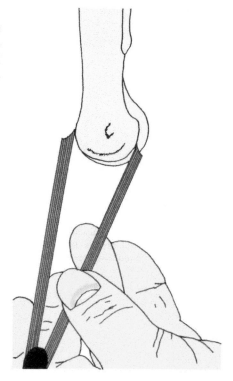

Fig. 3-22: The medial and lateral condyles of the fetlock joint may appear of similar size and proportion but when measured the medial condyle is always the larger.

THE JOINTS AS CAMS

Cams are used in engineering to control and change the direction of movement (Fig. 3-23) and that is exactly what the fetlock does. The pastern and pedal joints also perform similar actions. All of these cam-designed joints with their individual form are responsible for the subtle changes in directional motion. The distal or lower articular surfaces of the cannon, long pastern and the short pastern, form profiles with which to transmit motion, with the proximal ends of these bones forming the reciprocating followers. While the pastern and pedal joints are of a cam-design, they are less positive than the fetlock joint as they have the ability to compensate for uneven ground by allowing some uncontrolled medial or lateral movement. The mechanics of this type of joint are difficult to appreciate but for an example of how they work, we do not have to look very far.

The equine like all other mammals, ourselves included, probably evolved from fish-like creatures and it is because of this common ancestry that certain similarities can be found. In both the equine limb and the human hand, the same type of joints connects the metacarpal and the phalanges. To demonstrate just how these inter-

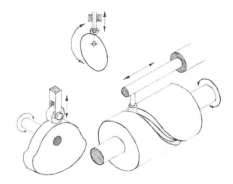

Fig. 3-23: Examples of cams. Cams are used in engineering to change the direction of motion.

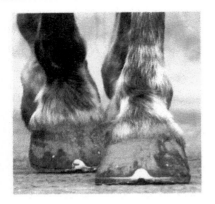

Fig. 3-25: As the fetlock descends, during progression (the hoof on the right), it shifts medially. As the fetlock ascends, during breakover (the hoof on the left), it shifts laterally, with the breakover occurring at the lateral toe area.

phalangeal joints work all you need to do is hold up your hand, preferably your dominant hand.

If we were to hold up our right hand, palm away from us we would see the tip of our first finger turning slightly to the right. If we then turn our palm to face us, the tip of that finger would tilt to the left and, finally, if we then bend that finger towards us it would once again tilt to the right (Fig. 3-24). Try it! This exercise demonstrates quite clearly that as the phalanges move, the relationship between the axes of each of the bones is under constant change. So, what is the role of this kind of joint? During the motion of the horse, it is quite likely that the lateral heel will land first and this will form part of the deceleration process. Then during the stance phase, force is absorbed and energy is stored as the body of the equine is maintained in a parallel line of motion above the ground surface. To accomplish all these actions the fetlock has to be a complex joint. It has to maintain its rigidity in order to support its load but at the same time be dynamic enough to control the backward/forward motion which creates the subtle changes between the distal bones that are needed to maintain the hoof's location beneath the equine's centre of gravity. At breakover, the dynamics of the joint are once again revealed as the wear on the shoes can identify, with the normal horse breaking over at the lateral aspect of the toe (Fig. 3-25).

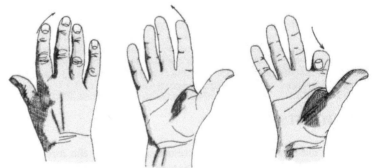

Fig. 3-24: A demonstration of how ginglymus joints control the direction of movement.

If we were to hold up our right hand, palm away from us, we would see the tip of our first finger turning slightly to the right. If we then turn our palm to face us, the tip of that finger would tilt to the left and, finally, if we then bend that finger towards us it would once again tilt to the right. These same mechanics form the distal joints of the equine limb.

THE ESSENCE OF FARRIERY

Outlined within this chapter is a description of the events that take place, with extreme rapidity, while the hoof is bearing weight during the act of progression. Even with a whole range of modern equipment, it would be impossible that a complete picture of what takes place for each and every individual could emerge. However, the information used to support this text is based entirely upon empirical evidence extracted from reliable experiments and wide-ranging experience. Footfall has attracted discussion for a long time and some theories have changed but throughout, there has been a consistent recognition that farriery, hoof trimming and shoeing, can and does make a significant difference. The real problem we face is not about recognising that farriery can make a positive difference but in understanding what that positive difference actually is.

BIBLIOGRAPHY

'If you take ideas from one source it's called plagiarism. When you take ideas from five its called research'

Axe, J. W., *The Horse, its treatment in Health and Disease* (Gresham Publishing Company Co. London, 1905)

Back, W., Clayton, H. M., *Equine Locomotion* (Harcourt Publishers Ltd 2001)

Clayton, H. M., 'Practical aspects of the equine gait analysis' (*The Fourth International Farriery and Lameness seminar* 1994 Handbook, p.9-11)

Craig, J.J., Craig, M.F., *Hoof and Bone Morphology of the Equine Digit: Challenges to some common beliefs* (EponaShoe Inc.) http://www.eponashoe.com/Documents/Morphology.htm (Access March 2007)

Gill, D. W., 'Hoof Balance: A working Farrier's Interpretation', *1st UK Farriery Convention Handbook* (Equine Veterinary Journal Ltd, 2001, p.59-60)

Gray, H., *Gray's Anatomy* (Bounty Books: New York, 1977)

Hickman, J., Humphrey, M., *Hickman's Farriery* (J. A. Allen & Co. Ltd, 1988)

Johnston, C., Back, W., Science: Overview; Hoof ground interaction: when biomechanical stimuli challenge the tissues of the distal limb, *Equine Veterinary Journal* 2007, 38, 634-641

Lardner, D., *Hand-book of Natural Philosophy* (Walton and Maberly, 1855)

Molian, S., *The design of cam mechanisms and linkages* (Constable & Company Ltd, 1968)

Parks, A., *In-depth: Palmar Foot Pain: Structure and Function of the Equine Digit in Relation to Palmar Foot Pain* (AAEP Proceedings / Vol. 52 / 2006, p188-187)

Wilson, A. M., Watson, J. C., Lichtwark, G. A., 'A catapult action for rapid limb protraction', *Nature* (January 2003, p.35-36)

Wilson, A.M., McGuigan, M.P., Pardoe, C., *Lameness in the Athletic Horse: The Biomechanical Effect of Wedged, Eggbar and Extension Shoes in Sound and Lame Horses* (AAEP Proceedings /Vol. 47 / 2001, p339-343)

Wyn-Jones, G., *Equine Lameness* (Blackwell Scientific Publications, 1988)

4: Anterioposterior balance

IN PRACTICE

Hoof balance is the most quintessential aspect of farriery, and it is without doubt the most important procedure that the farrier has to both interpret and assess; yet it is a discipline that has been so often poorly considered. In fact, in the not too distant past, hoof trimming was viewed as being quite simply just something that had to be done before the shoes were put on.

Although many of those writing about the subject have acknowledged its importance, it is clear that they had the opinion that the majority of farriers seem to be less interested in this aspect of farriery and more interested in nailing on shoes. The truth is, unless you know what you're looking at, one trimmed hoof looks much like another one, so it is difficult for any owner to recognise just exactly what good hoof balance is. Another factor that has always played a great (if not dubious) part in the development of farriery is that farriers are usually paid according to the number of shoes they put on. This single factor may quite possibly be the most significant inhibitor of real progress in the development of farriery because it places the emphasis on the forging of shoes rather than the trimming or balancing of the foot prior to the placement of the shoes.

Good quality shoes that are well-made are easier to fit, and form the basis of a neat looking job. The making and the fitting of the shoe has always been a high priority for those within the industry and that is hardly surprising; shoe making is a great skill even the basics of which takes a long time to master. Consequently, farriery has consistently been judged either by the aesthetic qualities surrounding the forging and placement of the shoes, the cost, or by the disruption caused to the horse-owning public. Farriers have themselves even contributed to the perpetual climate under which they work by suggesting that good farriery begins on the anvil.

As farriery is a free trade that has focused upon quantity and aesthetics the real need-to-know fundamentals about farriery have a tendency to be overlooked. That is until such time when all three parties, owner, farrier and vet, have had to consult with each other over a lame horse. The real problem with lame horses is that when it comes to farriery, the person who has the least influence over the management of hoof balance is so often considered the one in charge. Vets do need to know about hoof balance but it is actually the owner and the farrier who are responsible for the condition of the equine's

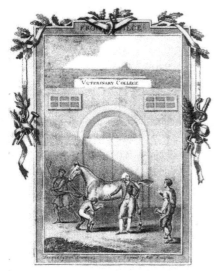

a L'afpect de La Verité
La Routine S'etoune, L'ignorance S'enfuit .

Fig. 4-1: The 'Frontispiece' to the book by Charles Vial De Sainvel 1793.

Professor Charles Vial De Sainvel, also known as St Bel, was the founder of The Veterinary College, London and featured here is an illustration which speaks volumes about the farriery industry both as it was then and as, some feel, it still is today.

Here within the shadow of the newly built Veterinary College, the veterinarian (the man in the long coat and powdered wig) stands directing the groom on how to pick up the horses foot. He is also explaining to the farrier what shape the natural foot should be and how best to shoe it.

Interestingly it was at this time that horseshoers became known as 'farriers' and horse doctors were to become known as veterinarians; until that time the term 'farrier' was in fact the name used by horse doctors. Horseshoeing, however, was still considered central to the welfare of the horse, so much so that the horseshoe and the tools used in farriery were used as symbols of care and aid to the horse; these can be identified around the ornate frame of the picture.

feet. Today's farriers are now being taught to understand and take into account hoof balance and it is equally important for owners to try to do so. By careful observation and a little effort to learn the basics, one should be able to acquire sufficient knowledge to be able to choose and then rely upon, a competent farrier. Essentially, getting to grips with hoof balance could make everyone's life, especially the horse's, so much more comfortable.

ORIGINS OF THE PAST

In 1792 The Veterinary College, London, later to be known as The Royal Veterinary College, opened its doors to its first four pupils, under the directorship of Professor Charles Vial de Sainvel, a Frenchman, known by his colleagues as 'St Bel'. Arguably, it may be that the foundation of The Royal Veterinary College can be traced back to a single incident and that was the death of the racehorse Eclipse. Eclipse was so named because of the solar event that took place on the date of his birth, 1st April 1764. This horse was legendary and had never been beaten. In fact, the horse was so famed and so important that at his death in 1789, at the age of 25, a post-mortem was carried out in an attempt not only to understand the cause of his death but also to understand why he was so successful. St Bel who was in England at that time stepped forward, as he was the only person in the country available who was considered qualified enough to carry out such an important task and his findings were later published. However, the real reason St Bel was over here was not to look at dead racehorses but to win support for his idea to set up a veterinary college right here in this country and the rest, as they say, is history. Unfortunately the Professor died in 1793, which was also the same year of the publication of his treatise, *'Lectures on the Elements of Farriery or the Art of Shoeing Horses, and on the Diseases of the Feet'* (Fig. 4-1). In his book, St Bel, the only man trusted to examine Eclipse, had this to say about judging hoof balance; *'we are hampered by not knowing the natural or normal shape of the hoof'*. Later Edward Coleman, renowned for his active involvement in farriery and his 'frog pressure theories', who had became the Professor of The Veterinary College after St Bel's death, wrote in his book of 1798, *'Men have attended chiefly to the shoe, and not to its application'*. Both those quotes could have been written yesterday and so hence the history lesson. It is in fact probable that more has been written in the English language, on the art of farriery, in the 150 years between 1750 and 1900 than at any other time in history. So to look at and understand anything about farriery one must start by looking at that time, the era of the horse.

'NO FOOT NO HORSE'

Most horse owners have heard of the phrase *'No Foot No Horse'*, a quote which comes from the title of the treatise by Jeremiah Bridges (1751). In his book, he suggested *'The best method to keep the foot sound is good shoeing'*. He also recognised the plastic properties of horn and how it can be influenced by the environment, *'The horses bred in Derbyshire, the mountainous parts of England and Wales...have good feet; while those reared on low marshy ground ...have commonly flat soft feet'*. The hoof's integrity is influenced by moisture; softer hooves change shape far more rapidly than harder dry hooves and hard hooves have less of an ability to absorb force or concussion. To bring that into perspective, wet winters mean softer more flexible hooves, mud and lost shoes and on the other hand dry summers mean hard hooves; hard ground and concussion- induced lamenesses.

In the 18th century shoeing was fairly primitive and in need of refinement and the evidence for this comes from the treatise by Strickland Freeman, (1796), who inadvertently provides us with the first real evidence to help both explain and understand hoof balance. Although photography was not a facility available at the time Freeman published his book, he commissioned some fine hand coloured engravings which can provide us with a snap-shot of the shoeing process he promoted and of the hooves that process created.

ANTERIOPOSTERIOR BALANCE

Anterioposterior balance, (AP balance) refers to the shape and conformation of the horse's foot when the hoof is viewed from the side. The same view is described in other texts as craniocaudal balance and dorso-palmar balance and even front-to-back balance. Many suggestions have been made about how to judge and assess what is good, what is bad and what is normal, but for anyone to form a truly rational opinion they would need to first analyse the influence, which create the hoof's conformation. Strickland Freeman (1796) gave us our first clue in one single picture (fig. 4-2a). The illustration depicts the style of shoeing that he advocated and the hoof to which it is attached provides us with the information which will help us to understand what that style of shoeing does to hooves.

Illustrated in the Figure 4-2b is the type of hoof which is commonly referred to as being of a long toe low-heeled conformation, with the anterior or front of the hoof set at one angle and the heels of the hoof set at a more oblique angle. Marks are clearly visible along the hoof wall and these types of marks are often considered to be a characteristic feature of laminitis and so have been frequently described as 'laminitic rings'. However, this judgement tends to be an incorrect assumption, as the marks in the hoof wall are as the result of hoof deformation, the compressed horn tubules bending creating ripples or ridges in the superficial horn. These compression marks form as the thread-like fibres, which make up the structure of the horny wall buckle under extreme load (Fig. 4-3).

For a long time now, hooves featuring a long toe low-heeled conformation have been recognised as being of the type of hooves which will predispose the animal to a variety of injuries; this type of conformation has also been associated with the development of navicular disease, a degenerative condition of the navicular bone. Although it has sometimes been suggested that this type of hoof

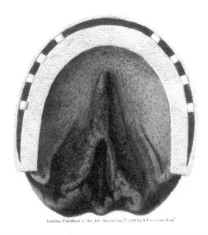

Figs. 4-2a: Strickland Freeman, 1796

Pictured here, above and below, is a shoeing style advocated be the author Strickland Freeman. It provides a clear and detailed account of a type of shoeing which as around at the turn of the 19th century. The detailed picture shows the shoe fitted wide but short at the heel. The heels of the hoof have very little support as the shoe fails to extend beyond the 'seat of corn'.

Below we can actually see the results of this type of shoeing. The horn of the hoof at the toe is at an angle of around 50°, whilst the horn at the heels is at about 20°. The heels having been crushed under the load created by the shoes being too short; compression marks are clearly visible; these are areas where the horn has buckled under the extreme load inflicted by the inappropriate shoeing style.

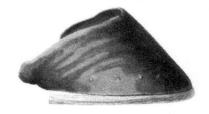

Fig. 4-2b: Showing ridges in the hoof where the horn tubules have buckled under load.

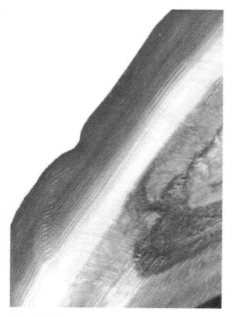

Fig. 4-3: Horn fibres buckling.

Ridges in the hoof wall are often visible; these ridges characterise the hoof deformation so often seen with laminitis. However these ridges also occur in hooves not affected by laminitis but are affected by deformation as a result of an excessive loading of the hoof wall.

conformation coincides with the development of this condition only, and that the hooves of horses with navicular problems will later become more upright, or 'boxy', as the development of the so-called disease continues.

Long toe low-heeled hooves have been associated with the causing of a whole range of problems and so, in the past, attention has been given to the shape of the hoof with attempts to change its form by raising the heels and shortening the toe. These efforts have proved futile, as in effect, this type of shoeing has been about rectifying a symptom instead of addressing a cause.

The system of shoeing which Freeman promoted must have continued and been in wide use for some years because that very same style of shoeing was illustrated and discussed in a manual by William Miles (1845) (Fig. 4-4a). However, William Miles was not promoting that pattern of shoeing, he was deploring it. The shoeing plan, which he presented, was one that supported the hoof more effectively by providing better length at the heels (Fig. 4-4b). He, like Freeman, chose to have exquisite plates made to illustrate his book and they show a much better, healthier hoof, with the toe and the heels of the hoof descending on to the shoe in a parallel angle with one another (Fig. 4-5).

Farriery today is the result of continued reflective practice, though progress has been slow. By reviewing the lessons of the past, the law of levers and the works of Freeman and Miles we find the proof that shoeing with adequate length reduces the effects of compressive force. So what about navicular, disease a condition, which has seen countless numbers of horses crippled or destroyed? Well, in November 1997 the Worshipful Company of Farriers issued a statement to all British farriers, '*Veterinary practitioners are now reporting reduced diagnoses of navicular disease. Leading veterinary surgeons attribute a significant part of this to the improvement of standards in general farriery practice over the last few years...shoeing and trimming to a horse's individual conformation*'.

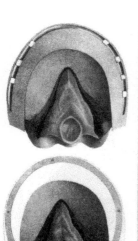

Fig. 4-4a: Featured left is the same type of shoeing recommended by Strickland Freeman in 1796.

Here William Miles (1845) uses it as an example of poor farriery; bottom left, Miles shows us just how ill fitting that style of shoeing actually was. The lesson we can learn from these examples is that, no! Not all farriers from the past did know how to shoe horses properly and that debate and reasoning can and will create a better understanding.

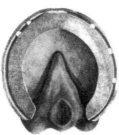

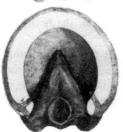

Fig. 4-4b: Here left is the style of shoeing recommended by William Miles.

The bottom example shows how his shoes extended over the buttress of the heels. He also favoured a unilateral pattern of nailing, with more nails on the outer branch and only one or two nails securing the medial branch. His reasoning was due to his belief that the hoof expanded during weight bearing and that this affected the medial side more than the lateral.

DEFINE IMBALANCE TO DISCOVER BALANCE

To discover balance, one must first define imbalance. Low heels, crushed heels, collapsed heels; all are caused by the two elements, shoe length and conformation. Too short a shoe will magnify the force imposed by the bodyweight of the horse both at stance and throughout movement. So if the structural integrity of the hoof is unable to support the horse because of unnatural or excessive loading, it becomes compressed. Compression is a force that reduces, so when the heels of the hoof become reduced, effectively the hoof at the toe will lengthen, which is why low heels are associated with long toes (Fig. 4-6a). When this occurs, the anterior surface of the hoof wall may very well take on a concave form. This is caused through the act of breakover: the tip of the pedal bone being forced downwards and backwards, while the horn of the toe is pushed upwards by the opposing force of the ground (Fig.4-6b).

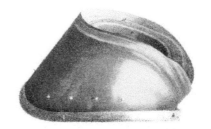

Fig. 4-5: An illustration depicting the style of shoeing promoted by William Miles, 1845.

This style of shoe provides good support at the heels and because of this, the angle of the hoof at the heels is parallel to the hoof wall at the toe, which is about 55°.

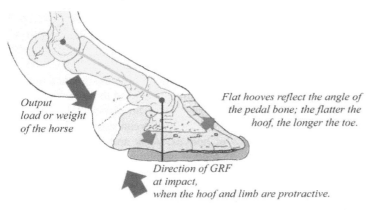

Output load or weight of the horse

Flat hooves reflect the angle of the pedal bone; the flatter the hoof, the longer the toe.

Direction of GRF at impact, when the hoof and limb are protractive.

Low/weak heels are exacerbated by shoes that are too short. The caudal aspect of the hoof can become so excessively loaded that the pedal bone will assume a more accute angle.

Fig. 4-6a: While the posterior half of the hoof is under load, the effort required to support the weight of the horse is augmented by the reinforcement/coupling of the flexible caudal regions of the hoof. Too short a shoe results in an overload of these regions (collapsed heels).

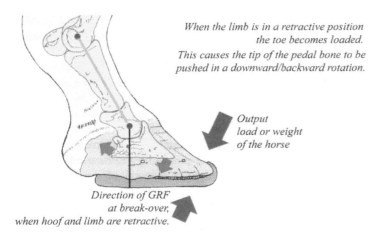

When the limb is in a retractive position the toe becomes loaded.
This causes the tip of the pedal bone to be pushed in a downward/backward rotation.

Output load or weight of the horse

Direction of GRF at break-over, when hoof and limb are retractive.

Fig. 4-6b: When the anterior hoof wall becomes loaded the toe of the hoof is pushed against the ground. Hooves with long toes and acute hoof angles are more liable to hoof deformation resulting in the horn tubules buckling and a further lengthening of the toe.

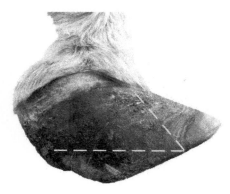

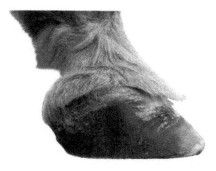

Fig. 4-7: Strong hooves can become imbalanced.

Strong hooves can suffer from imbalances if the hooves are not trimmed properly or regularly, or if the shoes are too short, or left on too long.

Pictured here is a donkey's hoof; the heels of this hoof are strong but they need drastically reducing. Effectively its normal base of support is so far forward beneath the pedal joint that the heel of the hoof is now acting as a fulcrum, causing both strain and pain to the caudal aspect of this animal's limb. Although this is an extreme case, the effects are the same to all equines. Horses with strong growth at the heels can likewise suffer if their heels are left too high, or their shoes are too far forward and when this occurs wear can be seen at the extreme heels of the shoe.

The strength or integrity of the horn plays a major role in hoof balance. A hoof made of good strong horn may have such integral strength that it can even appear to survive a shoeing style, which is less than supportive. However, sometimes appearances can be deceptive. Clearly weak hooves can be the result of inadequate shoeing but equines with good strong hooves can also be subject to farriery abuse either by the farrier applying too short a shoe or by the owner leaving the shoeing intervals too far apart. The law of levers is a rule, which affects all horses; likewise too short a shoe will affect the hooves of those same horses, but how? The weak-hoofed horse will suffer from crushed heels, collapsing under the weight of the equine but the strong hoofed horse having apparently survived those forces will shift the effect elsewhere.

Strong hooves that can apparently survive the forces of compression despite having been shod with shoes that are far too short will suffer damage elsewhere, in joints, ligaments, tendons and muscles. All of these areas can be damaged as the limb hyperextends, descending to become maximally loaded. At the point at which the fetlock would normally have reached a stage of zero motion, it continues beyond its usual range of limitations, causing the heels of the shoe to act as a fulcrum (Fig. 4-7). Now things usually work fine when they are allowed to work within their designated range of tolerances, however, it is when things are asked to do more than they are designed to do that damage occurs. So effectively, just as flat hooves can suffer from poor farriery so too can strong upright hooves, which is why both types of hooves, weak and flat and strong and upright are associated with tendon problems and navicular disease.

Conformation has its part to play in hoof balance. Things can happen or develop which are not the faults of either farrier or owner. Conformation is the result of the animal's genetic make-up and its interaction with the environment. To discover how that conformation affects hoof balance we need first to establish what is normal.

Finding a way to establish what is normal, what is desirable and what is the ideal has always been a huge and difficult task. Many have tried and although researchers have not always agreed, there are consistent patterns that have emerged. Therefore, it is these patterns that should be looked if we are to understand what are both the normal and the ideal, hoof conformation.

The years between 1750 and 1900 were years of discovery, debate and rationalization but the two great wars saw the decline of the horse and the closure of many businesses; farriery was in a decline. However, the 1960s and 1970s saw the horse returning as a leisure pursuit and with it the need for farriers to shoe them. With the old skills lost, many horses were subject to abuse through ignorance, so lame horses started to become part of the daily life of practising veterinarians. Then out of this scrambled beginning came a renewal of standards, better training, the thirst for new research and the Farriers (Registration) Act 1975.

Over the last thirty years, independent and isolated continuous research has been carried out and it is from this pool of information that the patterns needed to establish a formula to identify good hoof balance have emerged.

ANALYTICAL APPROACH

The first thing most people notice, when they look at their horse's feet, is the toe of the hoof. This should have a continuous form from the coronary band to the ground surface; a rule or a straight edge could be used to show more clearly any depression that may exist (Fig. 4-8a). If the wall takes on a concave form (a flare), it will be due to the downward-backward rotation of the pedal bone and the resistance of the ground surface pushing the toe of the hoof in an upward motion. It is usual and considered good practice for the farrier, when trimming the hoof, to rectify any deformation that has occurred by taking the foot forward and rasping the anterior hoof wall (Fig. 4-8b). The second most obvious feature but possibly the most important, is the heels. It is considered that the wall of the heel should run down from the coronary band at an angle parallel with the horn at the toe. However, we know that hooves that are shod too short may not achieve this because they have been compressed and become under-run but conversely, hooves that are relatively small compared to the length of the pasterns may also have a similar appearance. In both those circumstances, the law of levers plays a major role not only in influencing the hoof shape but also in determining the hoof balance of a particular animal. Horses with long pasterns and small hooves, by comparison, are unlikely to have such a regular hoof shape as those with short pasterns, relative to their size of feet.

Formulas have been put forward to both explain and to assist us in our efforts to recognise good front-to-back balance, particularly when it comes to choosing the length of a shoe. In the past, attention has been primarily focused upon the location of the pedal joint.

The pedal joint certainly does have a significant role in both stance and movement. Quite literally, the horse has to pivot around this influential joint but despite this joint performing such a central task, its functional influence upon the equine hoof means its location may not be in the actual centre of the foot. In fact, the location in relation to its surrounding hoof capsule will vary from one horse to another and it is because all hooves by their nature will be different, that a guide, which is dependent on the exact location of the pedal joint, may prove unreliable. Due to all the variables and complexities, any guide used to gauge hoof balance will always have to be based upon an ideal, and not the norm.

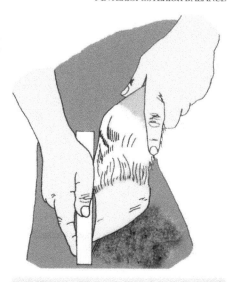

Fig. 4-8a: The trimmed hoof should have an even form from coronary band to ground surface.

A straight edge can be used to highlight any depression in the hoof wall.

Fig. 4-8b: To ensure the hoof has an even form the farrier will take the hoof forwards and rasp the anterior wall. This can be done by placing the hoof on the knee or by using a shoeing stand, or farrier's tripod.

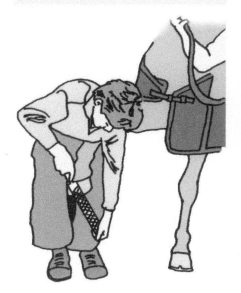

THE NEED FOR A GUIDE

The need for a guide is obvious and there have been many that have sought to provide us with their plans on how to judge good shoeing and hoof balance. Some of those ideals have come from farriers, some from vets and some even from owners. All of these plans are admirable but there has always been a consistent flaw with them all; they tend not to recognise that all equines are different. The mechanics of each horse are peculiar to that animal only; they are not all scaled down models of the same blueprint and yet conversely we can assume they all have similar needs (Fig. 4-9).

Fig. 4.9: All horses are not simply scaled down models of the same blueprint.

Featured here is Jack, a 17.2 h. Irish Draught x Thoroughbred, 6yr old grey gelding and Wicked, a 32" Fallabella x, 4yr old grey mare. Although both these animals are different in breed, size and shape, they are both affected by the same mechanical principles (Image: Mark Ellis).

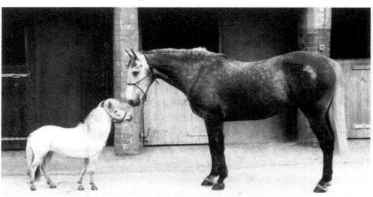

Modern thoughts have been based upon the location of the pedal joint, suggesting how much shoe should be in front of and how much shoe behind, the centre of rotation. Unfortunately, the variables are not always considered, such as the weight of the horse and its length of limbs etc. However when a collection of these plans are overlaid, a pattern does emerge, not one which is dependent upon the location of the pedal joint but one which considers the shape of the existing hoof.

Mathematics has long been considered the language of nature and everything around us can be understood and represented by numbers. In any given situation, patterns can emerge and from those patterns, graphs can be created. From these graphs and patterns, tools and techniques can be developed for solving specific problems or tasks. Mathematics permeates all aspects of our lives regardless of whether we recognise it or not, so the idea of shoeing by numbers may actually be more natural than we may first think.

Most of the shoeing systems of the past have relied upon the interpretation of the accompanying illustrations but more recently measurements and percentages have been included and it is from this wealth of information that a gauge can be designed.

A well-designed hoof model is an important tool, which can help to develop a common language or understanding between farrier, owner and veterinary surgeon. To design a hoof model or gauge it is first necessary to divide the hoof into equal proportions. Dividing the hoof into three equal sections is something which has been done before, Geraint

Wyn-Jones BVSc, DVR, MRCVS (*Equine Lameness,* 1988), suggested just that and other authors have taken that idea and penned the phrase 'posterior third lameness'. Both of those ideas or concepts have stemmed from the observation that roughly speaking the rear third of the hoof is without bone. It is this region which is the area most prone to compression and the area where most flexion occurs. The centre of rotation should also be considered, although the exact location will vary but in the design of any recognised model, it would have to be placed in the centre of the hoof, as in the 1987 edition of *Veterinary Notes for Horse Owners.*

Measurements for defining shoe length have featured high in the plans of a variety of authors and one such author (Don Birdsall, *Forge* 1990) has even linked the length of the resistance or load arm to the base or length of the shoe. Although all shoes need to be as long as possible there has to be a limit to their length because although lost shoes are a fact of farriery, we find that neither the customer, the farrier nor the horse likes them. Lastly, the distance from where the shoe terminates to the bulbs of the heels is an important one because that distance will grow as the shoe is pushed forwards by the growth of the hoof. As this occurs, there is a shortening of the effort arm that will result in the magnifying of the load, which it has to support. So when defining the ideal length of shoe we have to consider that primarily it needs to be long enough to support the horse but secondly short enough to avoid being pulled off.

Taking all that information as a whole, there is a simple procedure that can be carried out which will help anyone to create a hoof balance model from which an assessment of hoof balance can be made.

ASSESSMENT AND GUIDELINES

When it comes to trimming the hoof, an assessment is first made as to how much of the hoof wall there is to trim off. Depending upon the conformation and condition of the hoof, the heels are usually lowered to about the widest part of the frog. The amount of hoof wall to be reduced will be dependent upon whether the hoof is being prepared for the reception of a shoe or not. Once the solear surface of the hoof has been trimmed down in order to provide a sound base of support, the farrier will take the foot forward, place it on his knee and trim its anterior surface. The act of rasping the hoof wall should be considered a 'must do' because it is only by doing so that the hoof's true shape can be determined. In other words, the objective behind rasping the anterior hoof wall is to ensure that the hoof has an even form from coronary band to the ground surface. The initial first inch or so is where the horn is more compact and it is this area that provides us with the clue to determine the hoof's natural angle. The relevance of this aspect of trimming is not always recognised. However, the hoof which has been taken forward and rasped in this way, has a better chance of remaining both sound and healthy, while another, which has not been correctly trimmed but allowed to take on a concave appearance, will be abandoned to the forces and pressures, which will alter and destroy its form further.

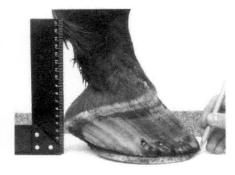

Fig. 4-10: Measuring the hoof to gauge an 'ideal' shoe length.

Featured here is a hoof, which could be described as having a long toed, low-heeled hoof conformation. The horn tubules at the heel can clearly be seen to be lying at a more acute angle than those nearer the toe. The old worn shoe was certainly too short for this hoof.

The novice farrier or the interested owner can develop a better 'eye', for gauging an ideal shoe length, by measuring either a trimmed hoof to help select a good fitting shoe, or a shod hoof to help assess how effective it may be in supporting the limb properly.

Measuring the hoof can be done by marking both the position of the toe and the extreme aspect of the heels on a piece of card. The distance from the toe to the bulbs of the heels should be considered the full and total hoof length, which can then be used to determine the shoe size and a reasonably safe amount of unsupported heel.

Once the hoof has been trimmed, a measurement of the foot can be taken and this can be achieved by simply getting the horse to stand on a piece of card. The distance to be measured is from the toe of the hoof to the extremities or bulbs of the heel. If the animal stands upon a piece of card, then it is quite simple to first make a mark at the toe and then another directly below the extreme aspect of the heel, at right angles with the ground. This can be done with the aid of a pencil (Fig. 4-10). The distance noted will be the full and total length of the hoof and it is this measurement, which will then be used to provide both the size of shoe and determine the amount of unsupported heel. These two lengths will be proportional to the initial measurement. To achieve this result, two minor calculations are made. The process of these calculations first divides the hoof into nine equal sections; eight of those sections providing an ideal shoe length, with the remaining section being the unsupported distance at the heel. The calculation is simple, first divide the actual length of hoof by nine, and then multiply that figure by eight. The outcome of these calculations gives both an ideal shoe length and a measurement that is relative to that length, forming the proportional distance of the unsupported heel.

The result of that simple mathematical formula is a shoe length that is relative to the size of the animal's foot (Fig. 4-11), a system that has in fact effectively been recommended by farriery authorities for in excess of two hundred years. Nevertheless, this is only a gauge and not a law; all hooves are different. Formulae such as the one described here should only be used as a model or gauge to help understand and recognise what hoof balance is. Taking measurements of each hoof is not a practical solution to assist with the farrier's daily judgements but by carrying out this process, with practice, anyone can develop an 'eye' to identify just how well any shoe may be supporting the hoof and limb it is nailed to.

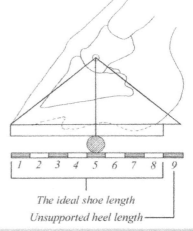

Fig. 4-11: A guide for gauging shoe size.

An ideal shoe size can be gauged for any horse using a simple formula.

With the full and total length of the hoof measured, two simple calculations can be made, which can then determine both the proportional distances of the unsupported heel and the shoe size.

The ideal shoe length

Unsupported heel length

First divide the total hoof length into nine equal sections (a calculator comes in handy); one of those sections will determine the unsupported heel length, whilst eight of those sections will then provide the measurement for an ideal shoe length.

Total hoof length ÷ nine = unsupported heel

Total hoof length ÷ nine x eight = shoe length

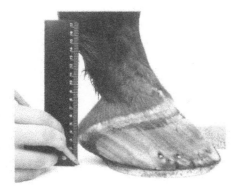

After assessing a number of hooves in this way, calculation may become unnecessary. Remember the essential measurement is not the length of the shoe but the amount of unsupported heel and this can be measured by an everyday object such as the handle of a hoof pick or one of your own fingers. Finding something handy to check against that distance, will prove useful because it is so easy then to monitor just how well the hoof is being supported throughout its shoeing cycle. As the hoof grows, the unsupported distance will increase and so too will the degree of force imposed upon that portion of the hoof; let that knowledge influence how often a horse is re-shod and not how much metal is left on the foot (Fig. 4-12).

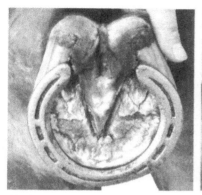 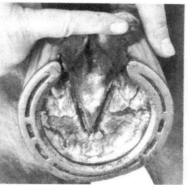 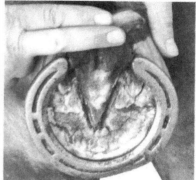

(A) Growth pushes the shoe forwards   (B) Gauging where the shoe should be   (C) This shoe is liable to cause damage

Fig. 4-12 (above): Assessing hoof growth and shoe length.

Taking measurements and working out formulas may not be a practical solution for the working farrier or the busy horse owner. However being able to recognise what is adequate shoe support, what is the ideal shoe length and understanding why should be considered an essential requirement both for the long term and the short term welfare of the horse.

(A) The shoe in this photograph is not providing the hoof with adequate support.

(B) This photograph illustrates how to judge where the heels of the shoe should be.

(C) Placing two fingers between the heels of the shoe and the bulbs of the heel will highlight just how far forward this shoe is positioned, too far forward and the shoe will increase the load on the heels and not support the hoof.

HOOF ANGLES

Hoof angles have often featured highly in any list of desirables and there are hoof protractors on the market, so that farriers, owners and vets can check hoof angles. There are also heel wedges designed to raise the heels or toes in order to 'correct' those hoof angles. The theme carried throughout farriery history is one of correction and the reason for that is probably because the normal has never been established. In 1802, James White published a book, which was to undergo many editions and reprints. His book was the first to illustrate what he considered the correct hoof angle of 45° (Fig. 4-15) but we know from Freeman (1796), that the hooves in his illustrations were

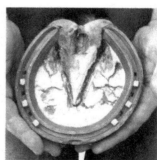

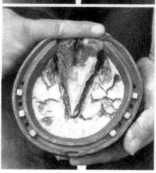

Figs. 4-13: This photograph shows just how far back a newly fitted shoe should be (top) and illustrates how we can best judge the shoe's positioning without having any special tools (bottom).

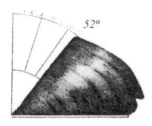

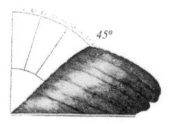

Fig. 4-15: It is without doubt the pursuit of creating both the 'correct' and 'ideal' hoof angles has inflicted pain and suffering upon generations of livestock for centuries.

However we now know that hooves, like the one featured at the top of this illustration are nearer to both the normal and the ideal, whereas the hoof immediately below recommended by James White is of the type we now call 'long toed/ low heeled.

of around 50° and that those hooves were hooves that were damaged by his style of shoeing. Miles (1845) on the other hand, recommended a shoeing style that he illustrated by showing hooves that were of an angle of 55°. Wild horse studies pursued by people like Jamie Jackson, Jim Millar and Gene Ovnicek, all from the USA discovered that the hooves of the feral horses they studied had hoof angles of between 50°-65° and of course, these had no involvement with man.

Anterioposterior hoof balance is one aspect of hoof balance that has been discussed for hundreds of years, and many of our current conceptions are drawn from the past. Various criteria have been suggested to determine normal or ideal hoof balance. The shoulder angle is considered to influence hoof angle and it has been suggested that the anterior hoof wall and the pastern angle should be in line with one another so that together they should reflect the angle of the shoulder and that somehow farriery should work to impose these theories. Many of these theories have originated without having any real foundation but more to the point have no real justification in their use.

The real take-home message of all the studies and research into hoof angles, pastern angles and shoulder angles is that these angles will vary from one horse to another. However, the common thread between all the studies into shoeing is that the best way to maintain a healthy hoof and limb it is to have the horse shod well and often. Healthy hooves would seem to have an angle of around 55° and those animals meeting this ideal, tend to have the pedal joint situated closer to the midline of the hoof than those of a lesser angle. Another clear message is to help avoid injury to the flexor tendons and the suspensory ligament ensure that there is as much shoe as practically possible behind the centre of rotation. This method of shoeing is also considered the best way to keep the hoof at its most favourable angle and that the size of shoe should be as long as or longer than the combined length of the long and short pastern (Fig. 4-16). Finally, those equines whose hooves are maintained at their optimum hoof angle will survive the effects of concussion better than those which have low compressed heels. And the best way to avoid crushed heels? Make sure that the shoes that are put on, fit!

'The best method to keep the foot sound is good shoeing' Jeremiah Bridges, 1751; *'No Foot No Horse'*.

Fig.4-16: Linking the base or length of shoe to the resistance or load arm (pastern length), was an idea first introduced to the UK by American farrier Don Birdsall in 1990. He suggested the size of the shoe, or the base of support should be as long or longer than the combined length of the long and the short pastern, and this concept can be readily achieved by using the shoe gauging system outlined within this chapter. Ideally, the base of support should always be longer than the pastern length.

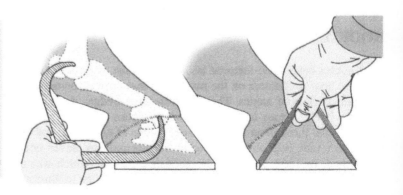

BIBLIOGRAPHY

'If you take ideas from one source it's called plagiarism. When you take ideas from five its called research'

Adams, O. R., *Lameness in Horses* (Lea & Febiger; Philadelphia, 1979)

Birdsall, D., 'Hoof Balance: Definition and measurement with respect of hoof balance', *Forge* (The Farriers' Journal Publishing Co. Ltd February 1990, p.7, 9, 12)

Clayton, H. M., 'Practical aspects of the equine gait analysis' (*The Fourth International Farriery and Lameness seminar* 1994 Handbook, p.9-11)

Colles, C., 'Hoof Anatomy and Function', *Horsetalk* (winter 1993, p.6-9)

Emery, L., Miller, J., Van Hoosen, N., *Horseshoeing Theory and Hoof Care* (Lea & Febiger, 1977)

Freeman, S., *Observations on the Mechanism of the Horse's Foot*, 1796

Gonzales, A. Z., *P. B. M.: Diary of lameness* (REF Publishing 1986)

Hayes, M. H., *Veterinary Notes for Horse Owners*; edited by Peter D. Rossdale PhD, FRCVS. (Stanley Paul, 1987)

Head, T. F. M., 'Open letter to all farriers' (*The Worshipful Company of Farriers*, 19/11/97)

Heymering, H., *On the Horse's Foot, Shoes and Shoeing* (St. Eloy Publishing, 1990)

Hickman, J., Humphrey, M., *Hickman's Farriery* (J. A. Allen & Co. Ltd, 1988)

'History of the College', *The Royal Veterinary College* http://www.rvc.ac.uk/AboutUs/Services/Museums/History.cfm (Access March, 2007)

Lupton, J. I., *Mayhew's Illustrated Horse Management* (W. M. Allen & Co. 1876)

Mansmann, R. A., King, C., Stewart, E., *How to Develop a Preventative Foot Care Program* www.equipodiatry.com (Access March 2007)

Miles, W., *The Horse's Foot and How to Keep it Sound* (Longmans, 1856)

Ovnicek, G., *New Hope for Soundness* (Equine Digit Support System, Inc., 1977)

Rooney, J., *Rings of the Hoof Wall* www.horseshoes.com (Access March, 2007)

White, J., *A Compendium of the Veterinary Art* (Longman, Orme, and Co., 1802)

Wyn-Jones, G., *Equine Lameness* (Blackwell Scientific Publications, 1988)

5: Odd but normal hooves ───────────

ARE ODD FEET NORMAL?

In a report, published by Northern Virginia Equine 2003, a veterinary practice in the USA set out to develop a rational hoof care programme; 50 horses were evaluated. The findings from the initial assessment illustrated that out of that study group 54% had non-matching pairs of feet. So taking that information onboard, if you are an owner, then there is a strong probability that the horse that you already own, or are about to buy, is likely to have hooves that are of differing sizes. Likewise, if you are a farrier or a veterinary surgeon, then the horse that you have been working on recently is also likely to have hooves which are different in both size and shape. In the past, these horses have had a tendency to be viewed with suspicion because of the long held belief that animals with different sized hooves are bound to be suffering from some sort of defect. However, the real problem that we have to deal with, is not with the horse but with our traditional concepts which continue to push the suggestion that all horses which are considered asymmetrical are either lame or in need of so-called corrective farriery. A rethink is therefore essential because if 54% of all horses have odd hooves then odd feet may in fact be normal (Fig. 5-1).

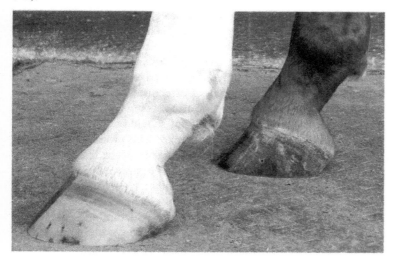

Fig. 5-1: A pair of odd sized hooves (courtesy Scott Gregory, farrier; Ohio USA).

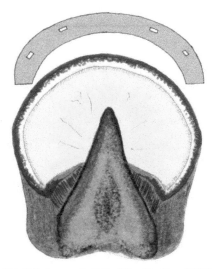

Fig. 5-2: A grass tip (after Wm. Hunting, 1899).

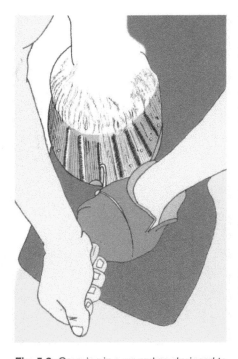

Fig. 5-3: Grooving is a procedure designed to weaken the hoof wall's structure, a practice that involves the cutting of a series of vertical grooves in to the Stratum medium. In the past, it has been used in the treatment of navicular disease and laminitis, although it is seldom used today.

TRADITIONAL APPROACH

Throughout the history of farriery, horses that have had non-matching pairs of feet have been considered to be suffering from a lameness problem. The logic behind this rationale is that many of these horses are either obviously lame or would appear to move in such an unlevel fashion that it would seem illogical to assume that they were not lame. These horses all characteristically have hooves that are dissimilar in size and shape, which in itself is a problem for the farrier; how to trim those hooves and simply deciding what size shoes to apply is a constant dilemma. At times, the farrier is often asked if he could literally pare down the larger hoof to match the smaller; a bit like pruning a bush. At other times the farrier may be asked to do the reverse and try to make the smaller foot larger and a variety of ways are attempted. Shoes are made and applied, all with the assumption that these hooves can be forced or stretched, to attain that which is considered desirable; matching pairs of feet. On the smaller hoof, 'grass tips' have been used to protect the toe from wear yet leave the heels unshod (Fig. 5-2). These are applied with the belief that this will increase frog pressure and therefore expand the heels.

The smaller hoof is generally considered to be the hoof with the problem and this is because as the horse trots it moves in such a way that the observer is likely to feel that the horse will be sensing pain. As the smaller hoof lands the shoulder will by comparison, appear to rise, suggesting a pain-related lameness in that limb. The apparently smaller hoof will be shaped quite differently from its partner, with more growth height occurring at the heels and the hoof taking on a kind of waisted appearance, with converging compression marks occurring midway on the anterior hoof wall. In fact, the appearance of that type of hoof has led to many authorities to describe the smaller hoof as being contracted, whilst the larger hoof is recognised to have gained its size through bearing more weight.

Traditionally, the approach to the shoeing of this type of animal has always been to make the hooves into pairs, with the most attention being given to the front feet. Both the shoeing and trimming styles, which have been consistently adopted, have all been designed to achieve this end. The smaller hoof or contracted hoof has not only had the heels lowered, but there are also accounts of where it has been recommended that the horn of the hoof should be uniformly thinned in order to make the horn structure weaker. This process is carried out with the idea that the hoof will then change its shape far more rapidly when certain types of shoes are applied which have been designed to encourage expansion. Grooving is another type of hoof trimming procedure, which has been traditionally recommended as a form of treatment designed to weaken the hoof's structure and so promote expansion (Fig. 5-3). The types of shoes which have been recommended to encourage expansion, are rather ingenious, ranging from the simple 'grass tip' to a 'T shoe' (Fig. 5-4). A 'slipper' shoe is another such shoe; a shoe which is fashioned in such a way to force the heels to slide outwards in order to create hoof expansion as the horse bears weight on that limb; and 'screw' shoes (Fig. 5-5). 'Screw' shoes are certainly a thing of the past, mainly because they're complicated to make. Again, the idea behind their design was that the hoof could be expanded by unnatural means, simply by turning two threaded bars united by a large nut; the shoe securely attached to the heels of the hoof would force the foot outwards achieving its objective. Today other much cheaper devices called 'hoof springs' are apparently used (Fig. 5-6). The hoof spring is a contrivance which may have gained its popularity within the US through widespread advertising. However, here within the UK, its use has been extremely limited and this may be because it is a procedure which has never been actively promoted. The hoof springs, as all the other practices outlined, are used with the idea that force will make the smaller hoof larger and if the hoof becomes larger then all will be well.

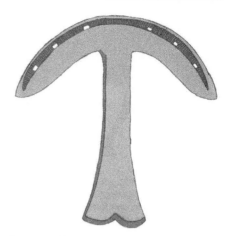

Fig. 5-4: A 'T shoe', or 'anchor shoe', designed to apply frog pressure, in order to encourage hoof expansion (after Dollar and Wheatley, 1897).

A RATIONAL APPROACH

With the possibility of over 54% of all horses having hooves that could be described as being mismatched, the probability is that they are not odd but in fact "normal" so if it is "normal" for horses to have non-matching pairs of feet why is it not desirable?

On closer inspection of the animals, which display non-matching front feet, frequently they can be observed as having noticeably different sized hind hooves as well; a pattern begins to emerge. If say the left fore appears more upright than its partner and the right fore by comparison looks somewhat larger and flatter; the left hind may appear in fact to be quite normal but its partner the right hind may seem just little bit smaller. In short, all four hooves are both different in size and shape to one another. Watching this type of horse, for even just a short while, allows another pattern to become observable. Many of these animals can be seen to favour a particular characteristic stance when doing what they love best, grazing. Tucking the smallest of their front feet beneath their body, they stretch their other limb out in front of them, the hoof on this leg being the flatter of the two. The hind limbs also form part of this pattern although this is not always quite as noticeable. This attitude of stance has long been observed and noted by owners, farriers and vets and this action is most frequently described as the 'grazing stance' but it has also been called the 'pasture stance' (Fig. 5-7).

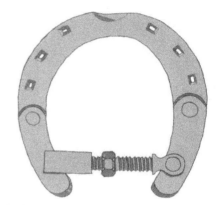

Fig. 5-5: A 'screw shoe', used for expanding contracted feet (after Dollar and Wheatley, 1897).

The equine is a herbivore spending much of its time grazing, in fact given the freedom to do so, the horse will spend as much as eighteen hours a day eating. Given that any action performed by any horse for such a long duration is likely to affect its body shape and posture, it would seem also likely that how the horse stands and behaves is going to influence its hoof shape.

Strangely, the behaviour of stance and its effects have not been prominently featured within the vast majority of veterinary and farriery texts. Instead, it has always been the hoof shape which has been consistently assessed and considered as being the cause of the animal's

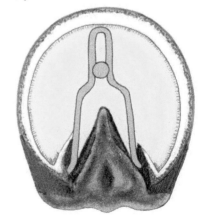

Fig. 5-6: A 'hoof spring' (after Lungwitz, 1913).

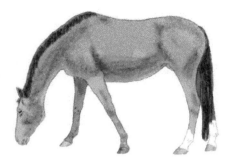

Fig. 5-7: The grazing stance. This describes the stance typically adopted by many horses as they graze, with one fore hoof being place in advance of the other, which is frequently placed behind the animal's withers.

stance along with any limb deformation it may have. In fact, for most equines the only time the animal's stance is closely looked at is when the horse is presented in the show ring. Showing is born from the desire of both owners and breeders to prove to others that they can combine their knowledge and skills to either acquire or produce the perfect horse. Whilst perfection is something considered to be faultless or correct, to the owner of a show horse, the concepts of classical conformation requires that the animal should project an overall beauty of outline, with movement derived from symmetrical proportion. However, our general perception of symmetry has a tendency to be based upon the concept of a mirror image rather than an overall appreciation of the fundamentals of balance, and it is this, which has been a problem, that has haunted artists throughout the centuries.

ART AND REASON

The quest for knowledge and understanding is a human characteristic and our need to know about the horse began at the time the first animal was harnessed. Treatises have been written about the horse for centuries, like the one by Simon of Athens (430BC), whose work was quoted in the ancient masterpiece *Xenophon on Horsemanship* (380BC). Aristotle also contributed to our present understanding with his works such as *On the Gait of Animals* (350BC). Acquiring knowledge is both long and drawn out with contributions being gathered from a wide variety of people and sciences and these are not always from the source which comes first to mind. Artist/anatomists have been, throughout history, one of the largest contributors to our knowledge of the equine. People like Da Vinci *Anatomy of the Horse* (1499) and Stubbs *Anatomy of the Horse* (1766) have through their detailed research been able to sketch out a clearer picture of not only how the animal is put together but of how it also behaves. Throughout the ages, artists have experienced great difficulty in depicting the equine in both a more natural and realistic manner. In 1779, Goiffon and Vincent published what is considered to be the first modern work that focuses entirely upon the equine gait, and this was a book published with the primary intention of assisting artists with their work. In fact, our knowledge of the equine has grown simply because of these people who have had an eye for detail. Artists, sculptors and illustrators probably know more about equine movement and stance than any other body of people.

For a long time artists and illustrators have made it their business to understand about balance and movement, and some knowledge of these two elements is essential to grasp any real understanding about farriery. It has long been accepted that the centre of gravity, or centre of the mass of the horse, is situated at a point just behind the withers, deep in an area within the animal's trunk (see Fig. 5-9). Though the exact location is a dynamic centre around which the body moves freely, in simple terms, its position would lie approximately somewhere under the front portion of the saddle, although that centre is in a dynamic state, shifting as the animal moves, leaps and stands.

THE GRAZING STANCE

The natural stance of the horse has failed to receive any real attention. The only time it tends to be noticed is when the horse is lame and when this occurs it is generally recognised that the horse will stand bearing its weight squarely upon its good hoof, while 'pointing' with the limb affected by pain (Fig. 5-8). In the natural and normal stance, the horse assumes a position which could be likened to a tripod; the hooves on one side of its body being close together while the hooves on the opposite side are placed much further apart. During the act of grazing, the equine's natural stance becomes more exaggerated with one forelimb stretched quite far out in front of its body whilst the opposite forelimb may be tucked further under its body, behind its withers (Fig. 5-9).

The act of stance may have escaped most people's notice but when it is realised just how many hours a horse may assume a certain position and link that to the law of levers and the plastic nature of the hoof, a new dawning of rational understanding begins to emerge.

To date, no studies have been carried out focussing upon the posture adopted by the horse as it grazes but studies have been carried out by behaviourists and nutritionists detailing how the equine spends its time in the wild. One of the most detailed studies undertaken by researchers was that of a population of Carmargue horses returned to the 'wild' after 30 years of management. These horses were allowed to roam freely for a period of 5 years after which their behaviour was observed (Fig. 5-11). Mares managed to spend almost all of their time on their feet with a colossal 78% of that time grazing, whilst their foals spent a mere 13% of their time lying down. The time budgets of other adults were as follows (Fig. 5-10); simply standing 28%, drinking 6%, lying down 5.5% and the amount of time grazing was a considerable 60% of the animal's day. Further studies have also shown that domestic horses have very similar time budgets to their wild and feral relations, in fact given free access to *ad lib* forage they will spend around 14-16 hours a day eating.

Therefore, in short, the horse spends the majority of its time on its feet standing in a very definite pattern. In the majority of horses the tripod-like stance, which they adopt while grazing, is alternated to a greater or lesser degree allowing the two pairs of limbs to mirror their partners. However, in a horse with a strong dominant side, a singular pattern of stance will emerge and it is these animals, which will display strikingly dissimilar pairs of hooves or mismatched feet. The main problem with those equines, which through their own dominant laterality acquire non-matching pairs of hooves and limbs, is simply that they are not symmetrical. There is nothing radically wrong with these animals; it is just that their hooves and limbs are merely shaped by their inherent characteristics. Therefore, owners need to take it

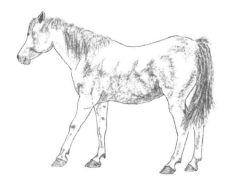

Fig. 5-8: The 'pointing stance' is associated with lameness, here the horse is bearing weight with the sound limb and resting the affected fore.

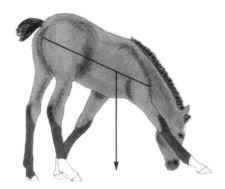

Fig. 5-9: The grazing stance is a natural stance free from manipulation. Here as the young foal grazes one fore hoof is place well forward, while the other fore hoof is drawn under its body and positioned behind the animals withers; behind the equines centre of mass.

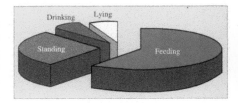

Fig. 5-10: The adult horse will spend a huge proportion of its daily time budget on its feet, feeding, or simply standing. Therefore, it is likely that those horses with a preferred grazing stance will acquire body-shape asymmetries.

upon themselves to both grasp and understand that these horses will never become symmetrical; farriers need to understand that these horses require their hooves to be managed, not corrected, and vets need to understand all of the above.

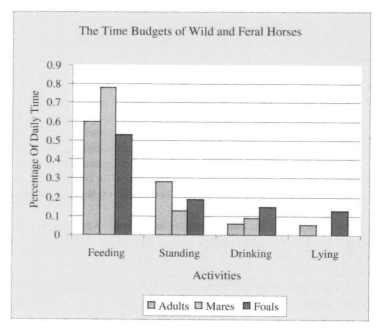

Fig. 5-11: The time budgets of wild and feral horses (after Boy and Duncan, 1979).

HANDEDNESS

Handedness is a concept which in farriery and veterinary science is rarely considered, yet it is probably one of the strongest influences farriery has to contend with. As a topic, it stirs debate but even when its existence is acknowledged, its effects upon the equine's conformation is seldom recognised or understood.

In 350 BC, Aristotle wrote his treatise *On the Motion of Animals*, he believed all things were predominantly right-handed and set out his reasons for thinking so. The belief was based upon his own detailed observations rationalised by reason.

Today it is accepted that approximately 90% of all humans are right-handed but the phrase handedness is not simply confined to the use of our hands. In a study which tested the limb dominance of 5,147 people, 88% were found to be right-handed, and a similar number, 81% were defined as being right-footed. The results of that study and other similar studies suggest that when we discuss handedness we are effectively talking about sidedness, or laterality, which is the preferred phrase chosen by some authors to describe these phenomena.

Handedness in animals is not an aspect that is terribly well documented or studied, however some scientific research has been carried out in order to measure the 'pawedness' of cats, rats, and mice. The results interestingly discovered that 54% of the study groups showed a dominance or preference toward one side or another; a result, which links very well to the findings of the veterinary practice, which noted 54% of the study group had non-matching pairs of feet.

Handedness or sidedness, in all animals including the horse, may easily be considered to be a disadvantage, merely from the viewpoint of survival. Handedness is effectively a form of asymmetry, which manifests itself not only in the dominance of one side of an animal but also in the deftness of that particular side. As a general rule, the ability to react and manoeuvre symmetrically is far more advantageous than having a higher level of dexterity on one side of the body than on the other. It would therefore make sense, that if anyone were to actually set out to design the perfect horse, which would move as efficiently as possible, then they would design it with pairs of limbs that were of the same strength and size. Unfortunately, the horse is not an object that has been designed, but instead is the result of organism subject to laws of nature and environmental changes.

The existence of handedness and its effects continue to be a matter of debate despite overwhelming evidence to support its existence. Even in humans, its implications have not always been accepted or understood. In fact, left-handedness has for many centuries often been viewed as being something of an affliction. Religious groups throughout the world have even looked upon left-handers as being cursed. Since the beginning of time, the left has long been associated with the dark side of religion with supposed close links to the devil. These ancient beliefs have long and deep-seated origins and have survived many centuries. It is no coincidence that sinistral means of, or on, the left side or left hand. Therefore, with the left being viewed as sinister, many left-handers have been encouraged, or even forced, to change or suppress their own inherent preferences. However, this type of imposed suppression has only been met with a limited success, with an estimated 60% of left-handers returning to use their preferred hand.

Genetics has been thought to play its role in defining handedness but to-date it has not been proven that a bias towards right or left-sided dominance can be predicted. Instead, it is considered to be the strength and not the side of handedness that is genetically variable.

THE LOP-SIDED ANIMAL

However, with regards to the horse, a number of authorities feel that their own observations suggest that the genetic component should be considered, at least when it comes to the incidence of unilateral flexural deformities occurring. As one veterinary surgeon noted, *'year after year, some mares will consistently produce foals that develop flexure deformities in the same limb'*.

Acquired unilateral flexural deformities occur, as the name suggests, after birth and are usually considered to develop at some

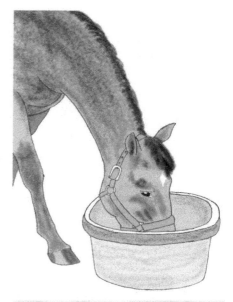

Fig. 5-12: Handedness studies, to-date, have been extremely limited, however there is one simple test that has been devised which can help determine the handedness of any horse. This user-friendly procedure has been used by a number of research groups and can be easily replicated by anyone, as it involves no special facilities and only takes a few minutes. The test, not surprisingly, is simply a monitoring of the grazing pattern but under some controlled conditions.

1. Place a bucket of feed at a distance of about 5m away from the horse.
2. Then allow the horse to approach the feed.
3. As the horse begins to feed note its grazing pattern (which forelimb is stretched out)
4. Repeat the test twice more.

The results have not been considered conclusive but one study found that around 50% of horses had a right side bias, 40% showed a preference to the left, while the remaining 10% were considered either indeterminable, or ambidextrous.

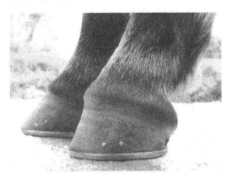

Fig. 5-13: The hooves of a 30-week-old foal that acquired 'mismatched' hooves, developed through an inherent singular grazing pattern.

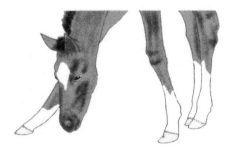

Fig. 5-14: A typical grazing posture adopted by young foals, as they stretch out their limbs, in order to reach the ground.

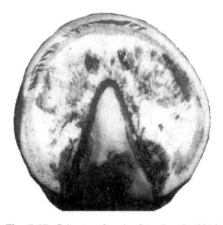

Fig. 5-15: Grit can often be found embedded in the toe region of the smaller, upright, hoof. This occurs in the un-pigmented horn where the Stratum medium merges with the Stratum internum; lameness is frequent.

stage between two and six months of age. This diagnosed condition affects one limb and is sometimes referred to as 'grass-foot syndrome' (Fig. 5-13). It occurs with the development of an upright narrow hoof on one forelimb whilst the hoof on the other forelimb becomes flat and low heeled. This symptomatic hoof combination has also been linked by a number of vets to the way the animal habitually stands; with one foot being placed well forward, overloading the heels and the other hoof placed under the body, compressing the toe (Fig. 5-14). As this type of stance is of such a singular repeated pattern, with the same hooves adopting the same positions during stance, the narrower upright hoof has a tendency to become worn at the toe. The result of this wear is often bruising at the toe as the hoof is sandwiched between the weight of the animal and the ground surface. More frequently than not, this localised damage is accompanied with the presence of small stones which can be found embedded into the hoof (Fig.5-15). These small stones or gravel particles, which have been compressed into the sole or white line, often lead to abscesses. It is now fast becoming the opinion of a growing number of authorities that this area of localised hoof damage is itself considered to initiate a pain related flexure withdrawal reflex, whilst causing the flexor muscles controlling the tendon to contract. As this process takes place, it is then that the foal's pattern of stance will noticeably change and the stance known as the pointing stance will be preferred.

The cause of this deformity is still widely considered elusive although genetics are considered by many to play the principal role in its development. However, taking on board an overall view of this deformity, reason would suggest that the trigger to this cycle of events is likely to be the strong dominance of one side of the animal, coupled with a failure to both recognise and manage such an observable pattern of habitual behaviour.

The evidence of sidedness would initially appear to be minimal. Most horse owners are ready to understand and recognise that their horse will have a definite or preferred way of moving, although not many of those same owners will probably know enough to appreciate that those tendencies which are both identifiable and inherent are the main forces responsible for shaping their equine's hooves. In fact, how their horse stands is likely to prove indicative not only of its foot shape but may also help to demonstrate to the observer which leg is its preferred lead; a clue that will then serve to illustrate which is its dominant side. Just as the grazing posture will be our first clue in identifying handedness, it should also be considered our first real evidence of laterality in the equine, with the effects of the animal's posture reflected in its hoof shape. To understand more fully how this will affect the animal's movement, we will need to look again at the grazing stance.

When viewing the grazing stance, what can be seen is in effect a snapshot of the 'leading leg, trailing leg' configuration, a forelimb pattern that is to be found in the asymmetrical gaits of both canter and gallop. These two gaits, the canter and the gallop, are very similar in pattern, characterised by the same type of diagonal action. To understand the implications of this action we need to get a closer look at the hoof and limb patterns made by both of these two gaits and to do that, a study needs to be made of the evidence supplied by the famed photographic accomplishments of Eadweard Muybridge (1887). In fact, it is beyond doubt that it is his work and the work by Professor Etienne Jules Marey, a French physiologist, which greatly influenced the classic text by Capt. M. Horace Hayes FRCVS, *Points of the Horse,* 1893. Although there have been many others involved in this type of study, it is generally considered that it is these three which have become the source of reference for so many students attempting to understand the intricacies of equine locomotion.

MUYBRIDGE AND LOCOMOTION

Most modern research into the study of equine locomotion refers at some stage back to the photography of Eadweard Muybridge born in Kingston-on-Thames 1830.

Muybridge (Fig. 5-16) published his own works entitled *Animals in Motion* and even to this day, it is still the starting point from which all other research into equine locomotion begins.

His excellent photographs show the sequential movements of the horse throughout the various equine gaits, with some plates that even illustrate how the transitions from one gait to another are accomplished. The results from these photographs detail many aspects of motion to such degree that each phase of every stride is visible, clearly showing the hoof's position from the initial ground contact and the stance phase through to breakover and the swing phase.

Many consider the patterns of canter and gallop to be variants of the same gait performed at different speeds; the canter is a slower three beat gait and the gallop a four beat gait performed at a faster pace. The term 'beat' refers to the sound or the action of the hoof making contact with the ground, so the sound or the beat is related to the footfall pattern of each gait. When the footfalls of two hooves occur with imperceptible timing then a single sound or a single beat would be noted.

A gait is a defined sequence of limb movements, which occur during progression. During one complete cycle of limb movements, there is a stance phase, when the hoof is in contact with the ground, and a swing phase as the limb travels through the air. When the stance phases of two or more limbs occur concurrently, they are said to overlap and when there are no hooves in contact with the ground then the horse is said to enter the 'suspension phase'.

The canter and the gallop are asymmetrical gaits with different ranges of movement in both the fore and the hind limbs, with two possible footfall sequences, either right lead canter or gallop, or left lead canter or gallop. The difference, which defines the canter from the gallop, is that during the canter the stance phases of the trailing fore and the leading hind are diagonally synchronised and are noted as a single beat, whereas in the gallop, the trailing fore and the leading hind are dissociated, landing at different intervals, creating a four beat gait.

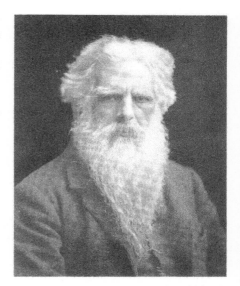

Fig. 5-16: Eadweard Muybridge (from 'Animals in Motion', Chapman & Hall, 1925).

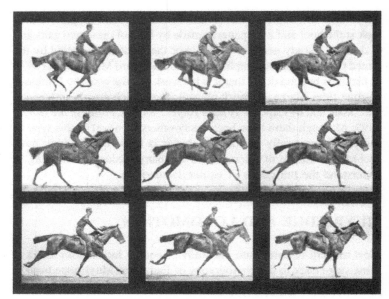

Fig. 5-17: 'Some phases of the gallop', taken from Eadweard Muybridge's 'Animals in Motion' (Chapman & Hall 1925).

The Gallop (right lead): During this asymmetric gait the leading forelimb not only lands at a more acute angle it singularly bears weight for twice as long as the trailing fore. The lead fore hoof is the last to contact the ground and the last to leave.

The asymmetry of movement, which creates the canter and the gallop, is not simply confined to the pattern of footfall; asymmetry can also be found in the ranges of forces exerted upon each hoof and limb.

CAUSE AND EFFECT

The hoof's conformation, which we see, is a direct result of physical force shaping and moulding the integrity of the hoof's primal structure. How the horse both stands and moves influences its shape, resulting in 54% of horses having noticeably differing sized hooves.

Through our own observations we can recognise that all horses will have their own preferred way of standing and we need to understand that this asymmetrical behaviour is quite normal; with those which exhibit a strong bias towards a particular pattern merely demonstrating their own inherent handedness, or laterality.

Handedness in equines is, just as in humans, a natural occurrence, not being the result of any illness or direct injury. Its presence is to be found in both asymmetrical usage and movement, which takes place between the left and the right sides of the body, which often results in an observable lateral dominance.

The asymmetrical gaits of canter and gallop can reflect a lateral dominance. The preference by a horse to lead with a particular limb has been noted not only by individual owners but it has also been documented in a study, which specifically looked at the '*Laterality in the gallop gait of horses*'. The study compiled by N.R. Deuel and L.M. Lawrence (1987) was described as the first scientific documentation of laterality, or 'handedness', in horses. The results taken from that small study group suggested a bias toward the left lead. However, the authors thought to draw no conclusions concerning the population distribution of handedness in horses, as they considered a similar study might well suggest a bias toward the right lead; their main conclusion was handedness exists and were happy that their study demonstrated so.

The objective of that study and indeed all of the studies has been to ascertain not only whether or not handedness existed but also to highlight the possibility that direct or indirect injuries may occur because an animal may have a propensity to lead with a particular limb.

Odd feet have all too often been considered the result of a problem; and if having a strong dominance of one side causes the owner problems then it is. The fact is, handedness exists. Limb dominance can be identified at a very early age and can be sometimes viewed whilst the foal is suckling and chewing at grass. According to Belgian researcher, Dr Verschooten of the University of Ghent (1992), *'foals are born with identical front feet that quickly acquire individual characteristics of size and shape'*.

Hooves conform to the forces that are placed upon them and it is the role of the farrier to ensure that the forces, which he may be at liberty to influence, are either positive or benign. How the horse stands and how the horse moves helps shape its hooves. At the canter and gallop, all the limbs adopt their own pattern of movement with the leading and trailing limbs and hooves contacting the ground at different angles, an occurrence that can be identified simply by taking a closer look at those famed antiquarian photographs of Eadweard Muybridge. Looking at the photographs of Muybridge and combining the information like that of the study by Deuel & Lawrence (1987), other residual effects of asymmetry can be noted, like the time periods spent on any particular limb during those paces. It would be difficult to understand why or how front hooves could remain the same if an animal prefers a particular lead, when at gallop it has been proven that the leading hoof singularly bears the entirety of the animal's weight for twice as long as the trailing front hoof.

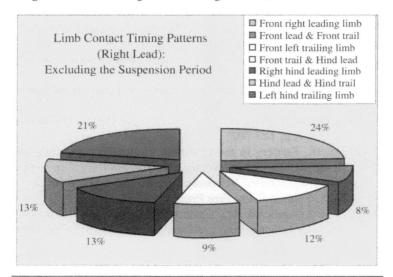

Fig. 5-18: Hoof contact timing patterns of the gallop gait (right lead), excluding the suspension period (after Deuel and Lawrence, 1987). The right lead fore hoof singularly bears the entirety of the horses weight for twice as long as the non-lead trailing left fore.

Of course, asymmetry results from not only how the horse stands and which leg is preferred at canter and gallop, but also how it shows and exhibits itself in the way the horse may be reluctant to turn to its less dextrous side. How the horse trots may also reveal some asymmetry and studies have been carried out to discover the incidence of asymmetry in Standardbred trotters and linked that study to performance. For the rider, the asymmetry in trot can be found in the way the horse will prefer the rider to sit on the inside hind leg, or the dominant side, again illustrating that the animal has a tendency to turn towards its dextrous side.

What farriery and veterinary science has to recognise is that handedness exists and that farriers and owners need to manage the condition together. Hooves need to be trimmed and shod, not forced into becoming pairs but sympathetically managed by redressing the balance and encouraging them to become pairs. The owner needs to be aware of the animal's predisposition and take conscious steps to encourage symmetry with the aid of schooling, making the less dextrous side suppler and stronger, and by monitoring its grazing habits. Having balanced grazing and stabling routines and ensuring, wherever possible, that access to feed and water is not at ground level but placed higher up will in fact, make a difference. Also ensuring that the horse is shod at regular intervals and understanding that when a shoe is lost it may not be the fault of the farrier but another indication of the equine's inherent make-up. Finally, vets have to appreciate all of this and remain both open minded and above all diplomatic, remembering that farriery alone cannot fix a 'crooked' horse.

BIBLIOGRAPHY

'If you take ideas from one source it's called plagiarism. When you take ideas from five its called research'

Adams, O. R., *Lameness in Horses* (Lea & Febiger; Philadelphia, 1979)

Aristotle: *On the Motion of Animals*, 350 BC. Translated by A. S. L. Farquharson (The Internet Classics Archive)

Axe, J. W., *The Horse, its treatment in Health and Disease* (Gresham Publishing Company Co. London, 1905)

Back, W., Clayton, H. M., *Equine Locomotion* (Harcourt Publishers Ltd 2001)

Boy, V., Duncan, P., 'Time-budgets of Carmargue Horses' (*Behaviour* 71; 1979, p. 187-202)

Castelijns, H., Farriery in the treatment of angular deviations and flexor deformities in the foal, *1st UK Farriery Convention Handbook* (Equine Veterinary journal Ltd, 2001, p.40-44)

Coren, S., *Left Hander* (The Free Press, 1993)

Deuel, N. R., Lawrence, L. M., 'Laterality in the gallop gait of horses', *Journal of Biomechanics*, volume 20, No. 6 p. 645-649, 1987.

Gray, E., 'Equine Asymmetrical Dexterity or, The Preferred Lead Syndrome', The Farrier & Hoofcare Resource Center (www.horseshoes.com) Access March 2007

Hayes, M. H., Points of the Horse (Arco Publishing Company, 1976)

Hickman, J., Humphrey, M., Hickman's Farriery (J. A. Allen & Co. Ltd, 1988)

Hunting, W., The Art of Horse-shoeing (H. & W. Brown 1899; Third edition)

Jurga, F., Hoof Research 1992 Report: Hoofcare & Lameness (www.hoofcare.com) Access March 2007

Lupton, J. I., Mayhew's Illustrated Horse Management (W. M. Allen & Co. 1876)

Heymering, H., On the Horse's Foot, Shoes and Shoeing (St. Eloy Publishing, 1990)

Mansmann, R. A., King, C., Stewart, E., How to Develop a Preventative Foot Care Program (www.equipodiatry.com) Access March 2007

Muybridge, E., Animals in Motion (Chapman & Hall: London 1925)

O'Grady, S. E., Poupard, D. A., Flexure Deformities in Foals (www.equipodiatry.com) Access March 2007

Springer, S. P., Deutsch, G., Left Brain, Right Brain (W. H. Freeman and Company: New York, 1998)

Stewart Hastie, P., The BHS Veterinary Manual (Kenilworth Press 2001)

SUGGESTED FURTHER READING

van Heel, M.C.V., Distal limb development and effects of shoeing techniques on limb dynamics of today's equine athlete (© M.C.V. van Heel, 2005)

6: Mediolateral hoof balance ——————

OUR PERCEPTION OF BALANCE

Most people's perception of balance stems from the concept that perfect symmetry, by definition, will mean perfect balance. With that in mind, it would seem both logical and understandable that our concept of mediolateral hoof balance should be based upon the ideal of proportional symmetry, with the medial and the lateral halves of the equine foot both being equal. This notion is seemingly so straightforward but if the concept of the ideal is that simple why then is it such a difficult objective to achieve and why, according to some reports, are there so many horses being diagnosed as having lameness problems associated with poor mediolateral hoof balance?

The reason and explanation of that view held by some authorities, is that it is poor farriery practices which are responsible for that lameness. It has also been suggested, though not substantiated, that 95% of all horses have some form of foot imbalance, which then predisposes them to injury, and that the majority of horses within the UK suffer from mediolateral hoof imbalances. It would seem also, that this problem is not simply confined to the UK; for example, in America mediolateral imbalances have been identified as a huge problem. One author concluded that not only improper trimming and shoeing is the most common cause of these problems but also suggested that it could also be identified whether it was a right-handed or a left-handed farrier that was responsible. Other authors have since retold this theory, describing how the right-handed farrier will have a tendency to rasp slightly more off the lateral heel of the left forefoot and rasp more off the medial heel of the right forefoot.

So by suggestion and implication it would initially appear that the majority of equine lameness may be due to mediolateral hoof problems, which may, as it has been suggested, be put down to the working practices of the farrier. Is this all too simple? Obviously the question of what is in balance and whether our notion of perfect balance is the correct assumption, is a complex dilemma and it follows that so too is the answer.

Poor hoof balance, according to veterinarians Olin Balch, Karl White and farrier Doug Butler, is without doubt a significant but inadequately investigated cause of equine lameness; they list sheared heels, chronic heel soreness, quarter and heel cracks, sidebone and deep thrush as potential consequences of mediolateral hoof imbalance. Gail Williams and Martin Deacon add further to that list by including degenerative joint disease, chip fractures in joints, fractures of the sesamoid bones and sesamoiditis. However, although all these maladies are considered to be induced by uneven loading within the hoof and limb, the three writers, Balch, White and Butler found the results of their studies highly intriguing.

'Attributing lameness to unequal weight distribution is disconcerting because anatomic observations, biomechanical bone strain studies, and instrumented force shoe trials provide evidence that considerable unequal weight bearing characterises sound, normal horses'.

DEFINING THE NORMAL HOOF

What is the normal hoof shape and how are we best to judge mediolateral balance?

William Hunting, FRCVS, a veterinarian who was the editor of the *Veterinary Record* (a periodical subscribed to by veterinary surgeons); an ex-President of the Royal College of Veterinary Surgeons and a member of the Committee for the National Registration of Farriers, wrote in his book (*The Art of Horse-Shoeing, 1895*).

'Everyone is familiar with the general appearance of the hoof. It is not a regular geometrical figure. Each of the four feet of the horse shows some peculiarity in form, by which a farrier can at once identify, a fore from a hind or a left from a right.

The front feet are rounder and less pointed at the toe than the hind; they are also more sloping in front. The two fore feet and the two hind should be in pairs. The right and left feet are distinguished from each other by the inner side being more upright, or, if examined on the under surface, by the outer border being more prominent'.

The asymmetry within the shape of the equine foot has been recognised and documented for quite some time, so too has been the suggestion that the forces placed upon the hoof have been somewhat less than symmetrical. William Miles, author of the book *The Horses Foot and How to Keep it Sound*, 1845, followed a plan of 'unilateral nailing', which he had adopted from a previous author and veterinarian, James Turner, 1832.

Miles, although neither farrier nor veterinarian, studied the hooves of horses over many years, observing those owned by others and monitoring closely the hooves of his own. He believed the hoof expanded as the limb became loaded and that this expansion occurred primarily to the medial aspect of the hoof. His observations on hoof shape prompted his reasons for a style of shoeing that avoided placing nails into that aspect of hoof wall which he considered the most flexible.

'The toe of the fore foot is the thickest and strongest portion of the hoof, and is in consequence less expansive, than any other part, and therefore better calculated to resist the effect of the nails and shoe. The thickness of the horn gradually diminishes towards the quarters and heels, particularly on the inner side of the foot, whereby the power of yielding and expanding to the weight of the horse is proportionably increased'.

100

Miles also noted and described corns, which primarily occur at the medial heel between the terminal junction of the wall and the bars of the hoof, he went on to remind and inform his readers that corns are not growths but in fact areas of bruising (Fig. 6-1). He concluded that corns occurred because of the shape of the hoof, the ill fitting of shoes and the load applied by the weight of the horse combined at times with the weight of the rider.

The asymmetries of the limb and an initial explanation of its loading can be explained and understood quite clearly through a relatively simple description; Haydn Price & Rod Fisher in their book 'Shoeing for Performance' state:

'The inside wall is fractionally more upright than its counterpart on the outside. This will accommodate the slightly larger amount of weight being taken on the inside of the leg since the centre of gravity of the horse is inside, or medial to the whole leg'.

So, with all this wealth of observation can we establish what the normal mediolateral aspect of hoof balance is? Well not exactly, as veterinarian William Moyer puts it:

'It would be safe to indicate that ideal foot balance could or should probably exist for a given foot on a given leg on a given horse but such an ideal is yet to be fully defined'.

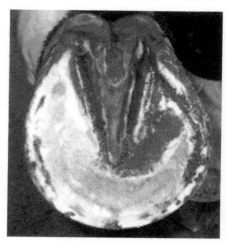

Fig. 6-1: A photograph showing the location of a 'corn' (a right fore hoof): a bruising, which can be seen on the sole, at the junction between the wall at the heel and the bars of the hoof (courtesy Gary Burton, farrier, UK).

At present we can only generalise and learn to identify hoof pattern models as best we can, nevertheless there is already one invariable sequence of nature, which for a long time has been thought to exist and that is, that the normal hoof shape is unlikely to be symmetrical. In America, studies have been carried out on a number of occasions, taking and analysing detailed hoof measurements; those results, not surprisingly, confirm that hooves are likely to be asymmetric. However, one such study revealed something really quite interesting. The study looked first at hooves taken from 95 thoroughbred racehorses. Of that group, 70 had been euthanised because of catastrophic musculoskeletal injuries, including suspensory apparatus failure and cannon bone condylar fracture. A further control group of 25 horses was also examined, which had died or been destroyed through unspecified though non-musculoskeletal causes. Unexpectedly, the results were to shatter the beliefs of many, highlighting that it was those horses which were affected by traumatic injury, which had the hooves that were the closest to the symmetrical, whilst those which had died through non-musculoskeletal causes, had asymmetric hooves. So, are asymmetric hooves both normal and desirable? Well the writers of that particular study concluded that *'trimming the hoof to perfect mediolateral symmetry may not be a sound approach to avoiding injury'.*

To find the truths behind the mishmash of conflicting evidence and to discover a sound approach to mediolateral hoof balance, we need to look closer at the conformation of the horse. As with the anterioposterior aspect of hoof balance the effects of stance and movement will also have to be considered. It is these two elements which will have the greatest influence upon the mediolateral asymmetry of the equine foot so it is essential to understand their

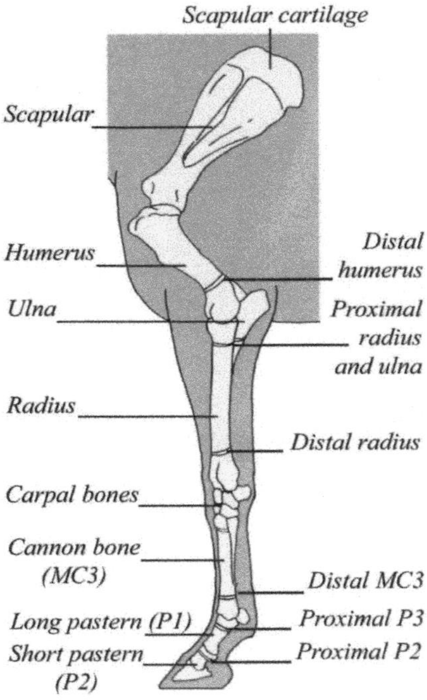
Scapular cartilage
Scapular
Humerus
Distal humerus
Ulna
Proximal radius and ulna
Radius
Distal radius
Carpal bones
Cannon bone (MC3)
Distal MC3
Long pastern (P1)
Proximal P3
Short pastern (P2)
Proximal P2

Fig. 6-2: The growth plates of the forelimb.

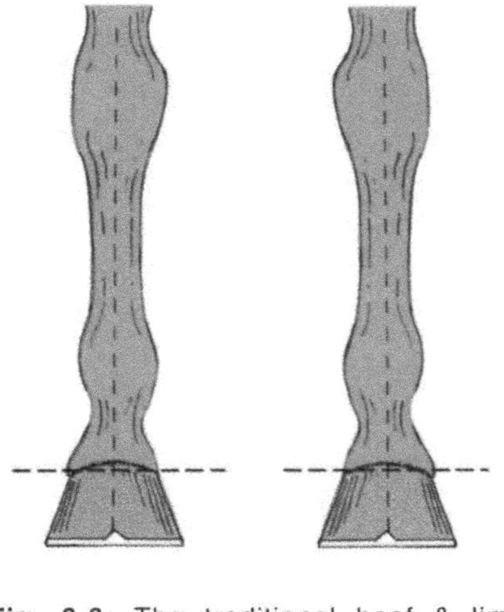

Fig. 6-3: The traditional hoof & limb assessment, referred to as 'static balancing', is based upon straight lines bisecting the hoof and limb.

effects if we are to identify an ideal hoof balance that is both normal and desirable for any individual horse.

ADAPTATION OF THE LIMBS

Conformation is, as the word suggests, the adaptation of the equine's structure, which was formed pre-birth and is a process which begins at birth and then develops through to maturity. The word is commonly used to describe the general outline or body-shape of the horse. The animal's conformation is shaped as the foal's body grows, adapting and conforming as it interacts with its environment. The term usually refers to the symmetry, size and shape of the various body regions, with each region being relative to one another. These points when judged as a whole combine to provide to the observer an overall appreciation of the visible proportions of the animal (conformation). Some attributes are considered desirable whilst others may be considered undesirable, depending on whether or not they may predictably have an adverse affect upon the equine's well being.

When the foal is born, its body's interaction with its new environment begins. The growth plates (epiphyseal cartilage), define the cartilaginous areas where the lengthening of the bone occurs; these areas are situated towards either or both ends of the long bones, which makeup the limb (Fig. 6-2). These areas of growth are highly important, as they are influential factors in the formation of that which is commonly described as limb conformation. Unlike the direction of the joint surfaces, the length of each bone on its medial or lateral aspect is not fixed and can be modified. Normally this process occurs as the limb lengthens and adapts according to the direction of joint motion and the overall displacement of the animal's weight during stance. In effect, what we are discussing here is structure and compression and their effects. It is these effects, which create conformation.

TRADITIONAL ASSESSMENT

Traditionally, limb conformation is assessed in two ways, textbooks tend to look at and describe conformation in a two dimensional manner with straight lines bisecting limbs and hooves with anything less than symmetrical being classed undesirable or incorrect. This type of assessment is a common translation of the process known as static balancing. The judging of static mediolateral hoof balance involves the horse standing squarely, with the farrier then trimming and shoeing the limb to achieve symmetry. The objective is to create the situation where the hoof and limb could be equally bisected by a line being dropped from the knee, continuing though the cannon, pastern and hoof, terminating with the ground at 90° (Fig. 6-3). This process is essentially, the same process, which in recent years been has promoted and involves the use of a T-square device.

A dynamic view of hoof and limb conformation is also sometimes described; this involves evaluating the horse moving to and from the observer. The hooves and limbs are assessed with the animal at walk and or at trot; the ideal is thought to be when the foot follows a straight flight pattern during the swing phase. The limb is considered imbalanced where the foot follows an arc, either inward (this is known as dishing), or outward (this is sometimes described as paddling). Another considered aspect of dynamic balance is the stance phase; the limb is thought to be in balance if the hoof lands flat and is then evenly loaded. As the foot completes the stance phase and prepares to enter the swing phase, the period known as the breakover begins. Here once again symmetry is thought to be the ideal, with many considering that the wear at the toe, which occurs during the act of breakover, should be central to the toe of the hoof.

Unfortunately many of these traditional views, no matter how long established, may not provide us with unquestionable truths and substantiated answers, To find those we will need to look further and examine the evidence.

NATURAL HABITS

Although symmetry has long been considered desirable, it is fast becoming recognised that symmetry may, in fact, not be normal, moreover, it may even be a concept which could be damaging if its principals are rigidly adhered to.

It is safe however to say that the majority of equine hooves are likely to be asymmetric. It is also safe to say that the ground surface of most hooves, when judging the mediolateral hoof balance, will not be at 90° to the cannon bone (or long axis of the limb). Both of these aspects are quite normal and both may, when closely observed, be visibly present in the majority of horses but what is the cause? Well, it is that simple prevailing force noted by authors Haydn Price (farrier) and Rod Fisher (veterinarian), the equine's centre of gravity (Fig. 6-4).

Habits of stance and movement are known to change soft tissue and those soft tissues include hoof, bone, cartilage, ligaments, tendons and muscles. Equestrians have understood this for centuries; after all changing the equine's body-shape, or outline, through schooling or training has always been both one of the effects and one of the objectives of dressage.

It is likely that the problems associated with mediolateral hoof balance can all probably be traced to the way the animal stands, as the limb will primarily adapt according to the continued, low-grade force applied by the equine's own weight.

However, the way in which that animal then moves can call upon the hoof or limb to compromise beyond a sympathetic range of tolerance, resulting in damage or wear.

Although there are no studies that are readily available, which identify the patterns of stance, we do know through documented studies, such as the *Time-budgets of Carmargue Horses* by Boy and Duncan, that the equine spends a huge amount of its time on its feet (*see chapter 5*). Habits of stance provide the reason and the

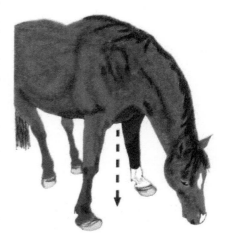

Fig. 6-4: The centre of gravity, also known as the centre of mass, is situated medially to this horse's front hooves as it stands grazing. The repeated low-grade force, applied to its hooves through stance, causes those hooves to be compressed (reduced in height).

Plastic deformation occurs because of the hoof's viscoelastic properties. The structures of the hoof provide shock absorption and energy dissipation. However, some of those structures are subject to a time dependent creep which means that they will yield or buckle under a prolonged load (change shape).

overwhelming force, which affects and shapes the equine hoof and it is this influence which is likely to be the root cause of most equine hoof problems. The resulting hoof shape determined by stance, may not always be the harmonious shape needed to ease and create fluid motion but may be the factor most responsible for the concussive damage so commonly associated with mediolateral hoof imbalances.

A FARRIER'S DILEMMA

Farriers for a long time have been aware that the hoof can change shape quite rapidly. Shoes which have become twisted and prised away from the hoof through the act of the horse over-reaching, will no longer support the hoof as intended; when this occurs it is generally referred to as a 'sprung heel' (Figs. 6-5). The hoof in these situations twists and descends where it is unsupported and so some farriers have thought to use this same principle with the aim of changing hoof shape. Bar shoes and half-bar shoes are sometimes used with one of the heels of the hoof (usually the medial heel), being trimmed in such a way that the wall at that point does not contact the shoe at all. This type of trimming is known as 'floating the heel'; this 'corrective' style of hoof trimming is applied so that through the influence of time and the body weight of the horse, the heel will forced into the desired alignment.

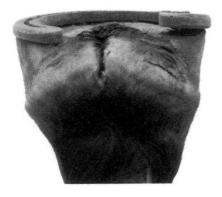

Figs. 6-5: A 'sprung heel', this is usually where a front shoe has been wrenched away from the foot by the horse catching the heel of the shoe with the toe of a hind hoof (over-reaching).

When this occurs the unsupported heel will invariably drop down to meet the shoe. This process, which most farriers will be familiar with, demonstrates the viscoelastic properties of the hoof.

Farriers attending hooves like this will sometimes leave the shoe off for a few minutes before refitting it. By doing this, the farrier gives the hoof time to return to its original shape.

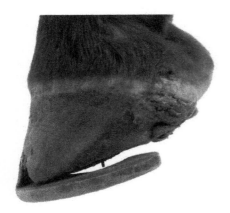

The problem we face (owners, farriers and veterinarians) is that there would seem to be as many theories about mediolateral balance as there are experts because, and this is where the confusion becomes evident, 'corrective' trimming has also been cited as a possible cause of mediolateral problems. Unless farriers and vets have a clear understanding of the main, if not all, of the elements, which affect hoof balance, lameness will be caused through the act of attempting to alter conformational defects.

After reviewing the evidence, the single most important message is that the weight of the horse and how it is displaced will change the shape of the hoof even after only a small amount of time. So how much time does it take to change the hoof's shape? Well according to one farrier, Martin Deacon FWCF, speaking on the video *In Balance*, hoof shape can change within as little as ten minutes of being trimmed. So, what about those horses with mediolateral problems considered to be caused by right-handed farriers? Well it would seem fairly rash to blame the farrier, who after all, is able to judge his work through the process of thought. It is more likely that those horses were themselves right-handed and that their hoof shape was primarily formed by the way in which they stood and moved; that process being an inherent automatic response and not the conscious process of thought used by the farrier.

So how can farriers begin to assess and judge mediolateral balance particularly as it would seem so difficult to define? Some farriers choose to follow the static balance theory based upon stance, whilst others choose the dynamic balance theory based upon movement but most recognise that both practices may create different results.

To understand why, is to understand the reason why mediolateral balance is so difficult to analyse and assess. Although those practices may seem well founded, the truth is, mediolateral balance is itself a paradox. Hoof shape is manipulated by the act of stance, which is a natural occurrence influenced by inherent behaviour but then paradoxically that natural hoof shape may not in fact be sympathetic to the way the animal then naturally moves; and so it is then when mediolateral balance becomes a paradox.

THE PARALLAX PUZZLE

To understand the process of what happens to influence the equine's hoof shape during the act of stance and movement we need to look at the three basic types of conformation. An understanding of the simple mechanics that affect those conformational types can be quickly grasped by initially focussing upon the forelimbs. The three main distinct types of conformation are as follows: Those animals, which toe-in, those that toe-out, and those that are considered to have an ideal conformation. Traditionally these conformation models are looked at in a standard two-dimensional approach; not surprisingly, this type of assessment can prove to be both subjective and at times appreciably difficult to understand. However, Dr Deb Bennett, who has a degree in Vertebrate Palaeontology and a wide based knowledge of the anatomy and biomechanics of both fossil and live horses, goes a long way to break with this tradition. Through her unique and informative accounts of how to assess limb conformation, she provides us with another dimension. She asks us not to evaluate conformation through simple two-dimensional lines but asks us to look at conformation in a three-dimensional manner, recognising that the limbs may very well face in a different direction to the rest of the body.

Dr Bennett explains how the limbs are set according to the direction of motion assumed by the elbow joint and that the humerus determines that joint's orientation. According to Dr Bennett, *the 'set' of the humeral head in the scapular socket is the ultimate determinant of 'toe in' or 'toe out' conformation*. She also writes, that *because the cleft of the frog is tightly attached directly to the bony column, its orientation will likewise reflect the plane of the forelimb* and this is why she asks her readers to look at planes not lines (Fig. 6-6).

So, what does Dr Bennett's interpretation of forelimb conformation tell us? It helps support and gives credence to the shoeing and trimming plans, which use the frog as a reference to determine the direction of the limb and therefore it should be a direct assistance in determining hoof balance. Her observations also help us to realise that the hooves may not face the direction of progression and this notion provides an explanation of why the wear at the toe, commonly described as the breakover, is normally towards the lateral side of the toe and not central to the toe. This is a pattern which can be identified quite readily as the farrier holds the forelimb in a position so that the cannon bone is in a parallel plane with the ground surface. With the hoof hanging

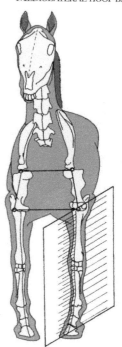

'Elbows out, toes in'.

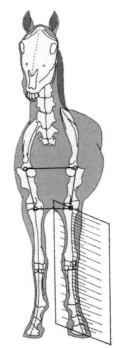

'Elbows in, toes out'.

Figs. 6-6: 'Think of planes not lines'. Dr Bennett suggests the positioning of the elbow determines 'toe in' or toe out' conformation.

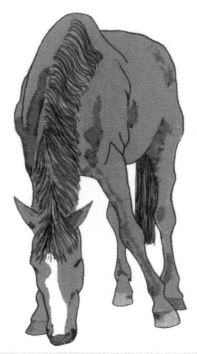

Figs. 6-7: All horses have a definite and identifiable grazing pattern, which will shape hooves. Prolonged patterns of weight bearing can produce deformation that may be defined as creep.

Creep is a time dependent response to the application of a constant load.

Below the hoof is shaped in response to its mechanical loading.

The recognition of creep is important because of the influence it will have on the biomechanics of the limb.

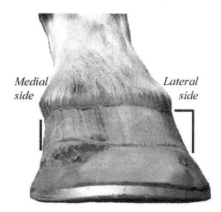

Medial side *Lateral side*

loosely, in those cases where a worn shoe is still attached, the wear pattern of the shoe at the toe, in other words the breakover, will also be parallel with the ground surface. Coincidentally it is this wear pattern so readily observed, which is indicative of the direction the knee joint relative to the position of the hoof. This suggests that the direction of the knee is not the same as the hoof and elbow but instead this joint follows the direction of progression. Could this be the reason why static balancing and dynamic balancing do not produce the same effect?

BIOSTATICS VERSUS BIOMECHANICS

How does the way in which the horse stands create hoof conformation? The simple answer could be biostatics but what is biostatics? The definitions would appear to be sadly lacking, as initially it would seem to be a fairly abstract idea. At present, in equine science, there seems to be little mention of the phenomena although P. Stewart Hastie MRCVS does make a reference to biostatics in his book *The BHS Veterinary Manual*. He describes biostatics as relating to the resting animal requiring an input of force to balance the output of gravity's force. Other references describe it as *'the study of relations between structure and function'*. Biomechanics is the science which brings the application of mechanical laws to living structures. It is a phrase generally associated with movement and has become a familiar expression to us all but there would seem to be little or no reference to the term biostatics, so perhaps that is a phrase ready for definition? One thing is for certain, how the horse stands can be linked to sidedness and asymmetry can be linked to lameness. The act of stance will shape hooves but is it ever considered that those shaped hooves may not then be totally compatible with how the animal will move? Put quite simply stance (biostatics), the action responsible for shaping hooves, and movement (biomechanics), may not always be in accord; those shaped hooves not readily adapting to the horse's way of going, farriery therefore has to be a practice designed to create harmony and balance.

So how does the way the horse stands affect hoof shape? Well the outlines behind the theory are already proven through the studies into anterioposterior hoof balance. How the horse stands and how it moves does shape hoof balance and it shapes mediolateral hoof balance in exactly the same way, which can then lead to imbalances affecting the comfort and well being of the horse. Those same actions and reactions experienced by horses that have so called 'mismatched' hooves are the very actions which also create mediolateral imbalances.

As the horse stands and grazes, it adopts a definite and identifiable pattern. That pattern then determines where its hooves are placed in relation to the animal's centre of gravity; the arrangement of each hoof's positioning affecting the force imposed upon its plastic structure (Figs. 6-7).

It is the limb functioning as a series of levers in opposition to the reactive force of the ground, which then moulds the hoof through the low-grade but frequently imposed forces incurred during stance.

All the joints below the shoulder and the hip are ginglymus or hinge joints; these joints, which are discussed repeatedly throughout this text, have great ranges of motion in extension and flexion but only have limited medial and lateral motion that is simultaneously synchronised to those actions. So, in relation to stance, all abduction and all adduction will stem from the shoulder and the hip.

Front hooves are the hooves which are predominantly identified as having mediolateral problems. This is because as the horse stands its front feet are placed quite a distance away from its midline or centre of gravity, whereas the hooves of the hindlimbs are generally placed in a much closer position to the midline. The effect that this has upon the equine's front hooves is to compress the medial branch of the hoof, which is an effect that, in turn, affects the lateral branch in a seemingly opposite way (Fig. 6-8). This is why so many authorities who use the T-square practice of assessment report so many hooves 'out of balance', the medial side having been naturally reduced in height. So where the hoof and pastern turn out from the fetlock the lateral side has a tendency to become more flared while the medial side becomes more upright. In the cases where the hoof and pastern turn in from the fetlock, the lateral side will become more upright while the medial branch will flare out. This in itself is not the whole problem but only one aspect because as the horse moves during progression the hooves are then placed close to the midline in order to maintain the animal's balance throughout motion. The result is that the lateral aspect of the hoof will make contact with the ground prior to the medial side (Fig. 6-9).

Lateral heel contact should be viewed as normal; it is probable that this forms part of the equine's deceleration process as the hoof contacts the ground. Anything that connects flat with another object will have to absorb tremendous shock and energy; have you ever belly-flopped when diving?

However, the problems arise when farriery management, in terms of redressing the balance, is not properly carried out allowing the hoof to become 'out of balance'.

During progression, viewing the horse in an anterioposterior plane, with the body facing the line of progression, it is normal, as the hoof contacts the ground, for the limb to be at an angle of around 84°-86°. Ginglymus joints accommodate for this; they are designed to allow the pastern to descend, with the limb proximal to the fetlock, continuing in the same plane while the hoof remains in a stationary position.

As the fetlock descends to become maximally loaded, its position is shifted medially, in relation to the static hoof (Fig. 6-10). This is essential so that the focal point of the limb, the fetlock, is in place to support the equine's centre of gravity. If the hoof is imbalanced and the lateral heel contacts much sooner than it should, it is then when torsional damage can be caused to the distal joints and ligaments.

Keeping the hoof within a tolerable range of balance and assisting the limb to function within its own peculiar comfort range is the benign act that farriery should follow. If the hoof is not periodically

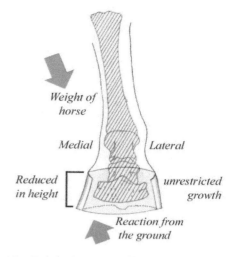

Fig. 6-8: During the habits of stance, more weight is borne by the medial branch of the hoof. This results in a deformation and a reduction in the height of the hoof wall.

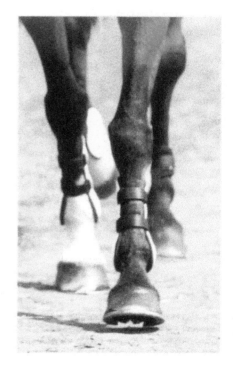

Fig. 6-9: During movement as the limbs converge to support the equine's bodyweight, it is normal for the lateral heel to contact the ground first. It should also be noted that as the heels are lifted during breakover, it is the medial heel which is raised first and the lateral toe region to leave the ground last.

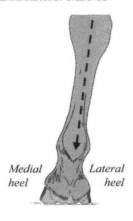

Medial heel   *Lateral heel*

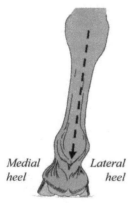

Medial heel   *Lateral heel*

Figs. 6-10: As the pastern descends it continues in line with the limb, shifting medially in relation to the static hoof.

redressed and this is more applicable if the hoof has a shoe on, then the hoof can become distorted or deformed. Where the hoof shape is altered from its ideal then the lateral heel will land too early, causing ligaments to strain and a greater load being applied to the medial heel. It has even been suggested that in the case of those hooves which turn out and flare toward the lateral side if balance is not redressed, a force greater than is reasonably tolerable will be directed towards the medial heel, causing the heel to be 'shunted' upwards.

Achieving and maintaining the individual's correct mediolateral hoof balance is of paramount importance but if subjective assessments of hoof and limb (static balancing), or footfall (dynamic balancing) cannot satisfactorily evaluate it, what guide is there for trimming the hoof?

BALANCING THE HOOF

So the question we all ask, how is mediolateral hoof balance to be assessed and trimmed? One farrier dissatisfied with the traditional assessment of mediolateral hoof and limb balance thinks he has the answer. Gene Freeze went back to basics and joined forces with Dr Michael Kirk, a veterinarian and fellow horse-shoer. They chose to study the feral horses at the Palomina Valley Mustang Station in Sparks, Nevada USA, where Dr Kirk was the federal veterinarian. Between them they examined over five thousand wild horses and concluded that it was incorrect to apply straight-line theories to crooked objects; horses legs. They recognised that although the bones within the limb work in synchronisation they do not share the same axis, so mediolateral hoof conformation had to be just that; hoof conformation and that it should be assessed in that way; by looking at the hoof. They decided that the direction of the frog was to be their datum line for hoof assessment as this is directly linked to the direction of the pedal bone.

Fig. 6-11: Gene's method for assessing mediolateral balance using the frog as a guide; this position provides the viewer with a silhouette, or outline of the hoof, which can be used to judge the trim (after Freeze and Harris, 1983).

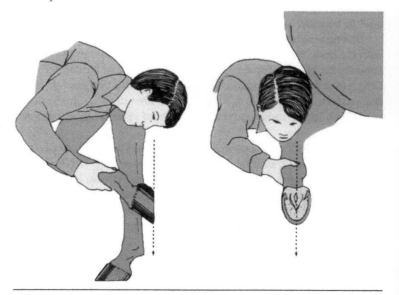

When looking at front feet, Gene recommended holding the hoof off the ground in a relaxed position with the cannon parallel to the ground surface, letting the pastern and hoof hang loosely (Fig. 6-11).

This he said permitted a true view of the bearing surface of the foot. From that standpoint, he suggested that you could position your head so that you could sight down the vertical line of heel, sole and toe, like looking down the sight of a gun but with having only beneficial affects. Having determined the direction of the pedal bone and looking down the hoof in that plane you need to look then at the medial and lateral hoof angles. By sighting down the hoof in the same direction as that of the pedal bone a clear outline of the hoof can be viewed (Fig. 6-12). Within this outline observed it is the first half-inch or so (1.5cm) of the hoof wall, from the coronary band to ground surface, that will reveal the pedal bone's hidden shape and from that view an assessment can be made about how much hoof can be trimmed off.

So, what were Gene's principals and objectives? Well not too dissimilar from other theorists, his trim is also an attempt to achieve symmetry, or as close to it as conformation will allow but his trim focuses upon the hoof only. Guides cannot be used drawing upon information taken from the pastern or the cannon, their relationship with the pedal bone and hoof is under constant change, so hoof balance has to be just that, hoof balance. Having identified the direction of the hoof a trim attempting to achieve symmetry between medial and lateral hoof angles is all that is required (Figs. 6-13)

A simple solution to a problem created chiefly through having an unclear, unreasoned, rationale.

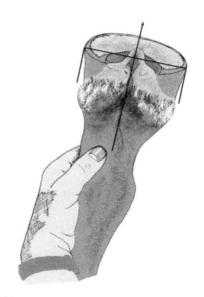

Fig. 6-12: Mediolateral balance.

Ideally, the hoof in balance will have hoof angles, medially and laterally, of a similar angle and these can be judged while 'sighting' down the frog.

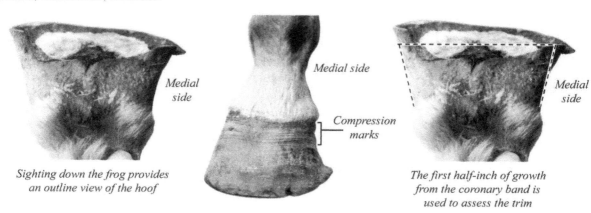

Medial side

Medial side

Compression marks

Medial side

Sighting down the frog provides an outline view of the hoof

The first half-inch of growth from the coronary band is used to assess the trim

Figs. 6-13: The principals of the trim.

- By sighting down the frog an assessment can be made, this view will give the direction of the hoof.
- Once that is established the outline of the hoof can be judged.
- The medial aspect of the hoof will normally be compressed and deformation visible.
- It will be the first half-inch (1.5cm) that will provide the clues about what angles the medial and lateral hoof wall should be. This is the area which follows most closely the shape of the bone within the hoof.
- The trim is made to restore balance usually by trimming more of the lateral branch of the hoof. This will place the pedal bone on a more level plane, which could be noted if an anterioposterior x-ray were taken.
- The correct trim will allow the joints to function normally, ease breakover and encourage straight and fluid movement, and above all make the horse more comfortable.

DISCUSSION

Our perceptions of perfect balance stemming from symmetry are not far from the truth; it's just that we, the experts, all have a different way of looking at the evidence. Straight lines cannot be drawn though limbs, the bones simply don't share the same axes and horses are not like tables and they do not move in straight lines

Hoof balance and the natural foot is a subject which has been discussed for hundreds of years. Within this volume, references are made to practices that date back to the 1700s; that is not to say that there is nothing new to add to our understanding. On the contrary there is always something new to add but by recognising past mistakes and looking afresh at old questions new truths can be found, that is what Gene Freeze did and we can all do the same.

BIBLIOGRAPHY

'If you take ideas from one source it's called plagiarism. When you take ideas from five its called research'

Balch, O. K., Butler, D., Collier, M.A., Balancing the Normal Foot: Hoof Preparation, Shoe Fit and Shoe Modification in the Performance Horse (Part 1); (*ANVIL Magazine*, September 1998) http://www.horseshoes.com/advice/balancingnormalfoot/balancingnormalfoot.htm (Access March 2007)

Balch, O. K., Butler, D., Collier, M.A., Balancing the Normal Foot: Hoof Preparation, Shoe Fit and Shoe Modification in the Performance Horse (Part 2); (*ANVIL Magazine*, October 1998) http://www.anvilmag.com/farrier/balancn2.htm (Access March 2007)

Balch, O., White, K., Butler, D., *How Lameness is Associated with Selected Aspects of Hoof Imbalance* (American Association of Equine Practitioners, 1993 Vol. 39, p 213-214)

Bennett, D., *Principles of Equine Orthopedics: Stance and Biomechanics for Every Horse* Owner (The Inner Horseman; newsletter of Equine Studies Institute © 2001-2003 by Deb Bennett, Ph.D.)

Bennett, D., *'Lessons from Woody' & 'True Collection'*, ESI Knowledge Base. http://www.equinestudies.org/knowledge_base/woody.html (Access March 2007)

Boy, V., Duncan, P., 'Time-budgets of Carmargue Horses' (*Behaviour* 71; 1979, p. 187-202)

Clayton, H., McPhail Chair Presentations http://www.cvm.msu.edu/dressage/articles/index.htm (Access March 2007)

Freeze, G., Are your horse's feet correctly balanced (*ANVIL*, July/August 1983)

Goody, P., C., *'Horse Anatomy; a pictorial approach to equine structure'* (J.A. Allen London 1983)

Mediolateral hoof balance

1. There is no real big secret about mediolateral hoof balance but each horse will be different.

2. The limbs cannot be used as guides to assess balance for trimming.

3. All the principal joints below the shoulder and the hip are ginglymus joints. What this means is the proximal and distal bones within the limb do not share the same axis.

4. During stance (biostatics) the medial hoof wall is compressed.

5. During progression (biomechanics), the hoof may land flat or lateral heel first. If lateral heel contact is excessive beyond that which is tolerable, damage to hoof and limb will occur.

6. Normal farriery is to restore normal hoof balance, as close to the symmetrical as possible but without the use of synthetic aids, instant changes do not mean permanent benefits.

Harris, S., *Gene Freeze: Are your horse's feet correctly balanced?* (Equus, April 1983, p 32-37; 45)

Hunting, W., *The Art of Horse-Shoeing* (H. & W. Brown, 1899, third edition)

'In Balance: Hoof Trimming for Competitiveness and Work', *A Farriers Guide to the Basics of Good Hoof Trimming* (Farriers Registration Council VHS video Parrett Productions 1999)

Kane, A. J., Stover, S.M., et al. Hoof size, shape and balance as possible risk factors for catastrophic musculoskeletal injury of Thoroughbred racehorses. (*AJVR*, Vol. 59 No. 12 December 1998)

Miles, W., *The Horse's Foot and How to Keep it Sound* (Longman, Brown, Green, & Longmans, 1856, eighth edition)

Moyer, W., Foot Balance *1st UK Farriery Convention Handbook* (Equine Veterinary Journal Ltd, 2001, p.61-63)

Price, H., Fisher, R., *Shoeing for Performance; in the sound and lame horse* (The Crowood Press, 1989)

Roland, E., Stover, S.M., Hull, M.L., Dorsch, K., Geometric symmetry of the solar surface of hooves of Thoroughbred racehorses (*AJVR*, Vol. 64 No. 8, August 2003)

Smythe, R.H., Goody, P.C., *Horse Structure and Movement* (J.A. Allen, London, 3rd edition, revised by Peter Gray MVB MRCVS, 1993)

Stashak, T. S., *Adams' Lameness in Horses* (Lea & Febiger, 4th edition 1987)

Williams, G., Deacon, M., *'No Foot, No Horse'. Foot Balance: The Key to Soundness and Performance* (Kenilworth Press Ltd, 1999)

Wood, R., *'Scientific Farriery'* (Tillotsons, 1928)

7: The crooked horse

FAMILIAR TRUTHS

Horses are very much like their owners in that they all tend to display some form of asymmetry, albeit in a wide and varied range of gradation, with the most common cause of any lack of symmetrical proportion being due to the continued habits of stance and movement. Although most owners are aware that their horse may have a preferred way of moving, this is a fact which unfortunately is not always fully considered.

However, the inherent characteristics displayed within stance and movement are without doubt, the most likely reasons behind any form of asymmetry affecting the equine's body shape, with the continuous interactions between nature and nurture being ever present.

Although handedness is fast becoming more readily acknowledged, it is generally recognised that the equine will also acquire noticeable forms of asymmetry through prolonged and continued practices, with many of those practices being often thought to be inadvertently introduced by ignorant handling and thoughtless management. If there is a possibility that handling and management can induce asymmetry, then controlled management and educated handling can, by the same assumption, help to produce the symmetrical horse.

The horses that have been described throughout this text exhibit distinct behavioural patterns, which then influence hoof shape, the most obvious one being the act of grazing, an act free from manipulation and therefore clearly inherent.

The grazing stance has a tendency to reflect the degree of asymmetry by which the animal may be influenced. It will also serve as a good indicator of which side will be its dominant or preferred side (handedness). The grazing stance reflects the leading-limb trailing-limb configuration (Fig. 7-1). The flatter hoof has its form acquired through a continued and prolonged low-grade force and has been recognised as belonging to the limb which assumes the role during the asymmetric gaits of canter and gallop, of the leading leg (Fig. 7-2). This limb has also been identified as having an apparently shorter distal limb, which is an effect that is created by the overwhelming act of compression. The limb which assumes the role of the trailing leg, receives the greatest compression to the toe of the hoof both during motion and during the act of grazing, and through that act acquires a distinctly smaller more upright hoof conformation than its partner.

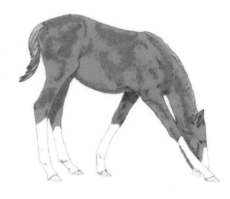

Fig. 7-1: The Grazing Stance is an act free from manipulation and has a tendency to reflect the animal's asymmetry and identify its preference to lead with a particular limb (handedness). In fact, the trailing and leading limb configuration can be seen to be identifiable within the grazing stance.

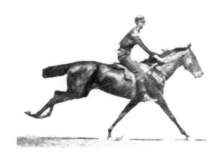

Fig. 7-2: The trailing limb and leading limb in gallop, taken from Muybridge's *Animals in Motion*. (Chapman & Hall, 1925).

FUNCTIONAL LIMB-LENGTH

Apparent limb-length is an acquired condition, which to date has not been scientifically documented. However, its existence is not so much questioned as ignored.

The equine's apparent or functional limb-length is a condition that needs to be clearly defined. Actual limb-length discrepancies occur rarely in humans. Statistically, present day research suggests that one in 452 people are afflicted with this disorder which is either congenital or as the result of injury. Functional limb-length, which in humans affects three out of every five people, differs essentially from actual limb-length in that under close observation each pair of limbs would, if measured, be clearly anatomically the same. The bones within each limb, of a horse affected by functional limb-length discrepancies, would be of correspondingly similar proportions, whereas with actual limb-length discrepancy, bone length would not be the same.

In the equine, the apparent limb-length disparities are caused by the functional differences of the preferred leading and trailing limbs, which noticeably stretch the palmar soft tissues within the distal limb. These differences, which can occur between the pairs of limbs, are acquired through the continued and repeated cycles of movement. As this continuous process of movement occurs, a responsive sequence of damage and repair takes place allowing the tissues of hoof, bone, cartilage, ligament and tendons, to adapt and lengthen according to each limb's normal range of motion. The undesirable side effect of the equine's asymmetry or sidedness which can be identified by the manner in which it grazes, is indicative of the way that it moves, producing limbs which are both effectively different in length and functional dominance.

LEADING AND TRAILING LIMBS

In the canter, which is a three-beat gait with the leading legs on the same side, the first limb to contact the ground of each pair of limbs (front and hind), within the definition of this particular gait, is known as the trailing limb. The sequence of footfalls within this gait is as follows, trailing hind, leading hind and trailing fore (landing simultaneously), and then the leading fore. At that pace the animal is both more comfortable and secure with his leading limbs being on the inside of any turn or circle. So if a horse is said to be cantering to the right, that will mean he will be more willing to turn to the right and in doing so, his leading legs will be on the inside of that circle.

The leading limbs and trailing limbs perform different tasks and functions. Although much evidence can be gleaned from the photographs of Eadweard Muybridge (1887) (Fig. 7-3) more recent studies have added to that evidence. Willem Back published a paper in 1997, which focussed upon the comparison of the leading and trailing limbs at the canter. He found that the leading limbs had a more forward range of motion (protractive) with the trailing limbs demonstrating a more caudal range of motion (retractive). This was achieved by the leading limbs having a far greater degree of flexion at both the elbow and the hip. In total, he found that the leading limb had a much wider range of motion; this allowed the leading hoof to reach out further than the trailing hoof. Another research scientist, Sloet van Oldruitenborgh-Oosterbaan, looking at locomotion during treadmill exercise, found that the fetlocks of the trailing limbs were more extended at ground contact and from that evidence, it could be deduced they would be more loaded during the initial ground contact and impact phase. In other words, they were more subject to a concussive force than the leading limbs, an assumption that was in accordance with previous studies using force plate analysis looking at mounted horses moving at the canter. One of the overall conclusions that researchers have come to, is that the leading limb is the swinging limb while the trailing limb is the more supporting, an observation echoed by other more practical observers who have likened the trailing limb as having the functional role of a crutch (Fig. 7-4). It is through these two very different roles of the leading and trailing limbs that through a continued practice of unilateral preferences that marked asymmetry can become a problem.

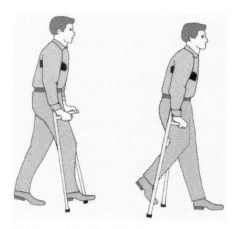

Fig. 7-4: 'The similarity of the use of crutches to the action of the trailing forelimb'.

The analogy of likening the functional role of the trailing forelimb to the usage of a pair of crutches is not uncommon. Emery, Miller and Van Hoosen, in 'Horseshoeing Theory and Hoof Care', 1977, make such a similar observation and owners and riders are also known to make such analogies, often describing the action of the horse as it uses the trailing non-dominant limb as a kind of prop. The trailing limb acts as a support whilst allowing the lead limb to swing forward.

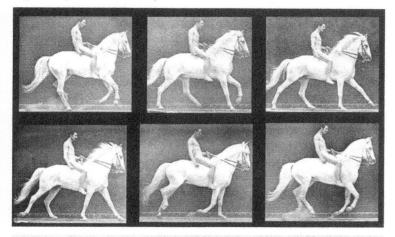

Fig.7-3: 'Some phases of the canter', taken from Eadweard Muybridge 'Animals in Motion' (Chapman & Hall 1925).

The Canter in this illustration (left lead): The trailing hind lands, then the trailing fore slightly before leading hind and finally the leading fore. The trailing hind is lifted, and then the trailing fore slightly ahead of the leading hind and finally the leading fore is lifted. When the trailing limbs land, they land at an obtuse angle compared with the leading limbs; similarly, when the leading limbs land they contact the ground at a more acute angle than the trailing limbs.

ACQUISITION OF ASYMMETRY

Repetitions of actions and motions are known to have a profound effect upon the human body, with excessive motion creating injury to soft tissues and joints. However, the continued adoption of a singular stance is also known to be equally demanding, creating overuse of the same muscles and displacing bone and soft tissue. Static posture is something that theoretically needs to be continuously changed, not only because to maintain a singular posture is extremely tiring, but also damaging. Therefore, if symmetrical proportion and dexterity are to be encouraged and developed, then an equally shared proportional usage of the limbs is required.

In people, sidedness and in particular the habit of bearing more weight on one particular leg when standing, can lead to an adaptation of the spine and pelvis, creating functional limb-length discrepancies. Moreover, where the eye and limb dominances are on the same side of the body, the centre of gravity is located towards the dominant side causing the body to twist away from its symmetrical alignment. This scenario is one that is known to affect runners who are strongly one-sided with their weight being more focussed towards their dominant side; this results in a tendency to veer away from a chosen line. Another effect experienced by runners is the feeling that one foot may impact the ground with a greater force than the other, which in itself is an act that may also be linked to apparent limb-length.

Although the effects described are related to the apparent limb-lengths in humans and the cause and effect of apparent limb-length is not consistently documented, there are a growing number of authorities within the equine world that believe its existence is to be found within the majority of horses. Tony Gonzales and Dr. Deb Bennett have both conducted extensive research into this subject and although at first glance there may appear to be some inconsistencies within their work, there is a strong theme that runs throughout and the evidence supporting limb-length discrepancies is clearly overwhelming. However, it needs to be remembered that there are wide and various ranges of asymmetry or sidedness. Therefore, if your horse or the horse that you have just been looking at does not appear to fit into the most obvious patterns of asymmetry, consider it the exception that proves the rule, and the rule is, all horses are different.

REVIEWING THE EVIDENCE

So, what is the most common and most noticeable form of asymmetry we are likely to see? Well according to Dr. Deb Bennett most horses display odd sized front feet, with one foot being noticeably larger and flatter, with the other being smaller and 'clubby' looking. She feels that where these odd feet are more apparent, it is the right one which tends to be the larger, an observation that concurs with the studies carried out by army farrier Ivon Bell FWCF.

Between October 1992 to June 1993, Ivon Bell carried out a study of 150 horses, the results of which focussed upon hoof size, hoof angles, limb lameness, injuries and shoe wear.

Like Dr. Deb Bennett, he too found that in 25% of those horses he looked at, the right front foot was larger, while 17% had larger left hooves and in 58%, he found no discernible disparity in hoof size at all. He also added weight to his observation, with an addendum to his study, noting that during his experiences in Hong Kong while working with retired racehorses, he found that these had a high propensity to having larger right front feet (Fig. 7-5).

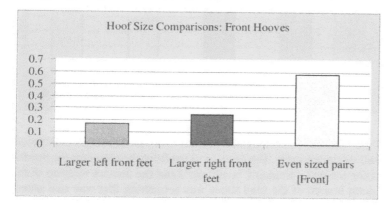

Fig. 7-5: British Army: hoof size comparisons, from a study looking at 150 horses and measuring their hoof width (front). The study showed a significant bias to the right fore being the larger (Ivon Bell, 1994).

He also added that these were trained and raced on tight oval shaped tracks, consistently being asked to run in a clockwise direction. The question raised in this one single observation was, did these animals develop larger right front hooves because of what they were asked to do, or were they selected for those tracks because they had the natural ability to perform well galloping with the right lead? One thing was clear however, whichever front hoof was found to be the larger, the hoof angle was more acute than the angle of the smaller hoof.

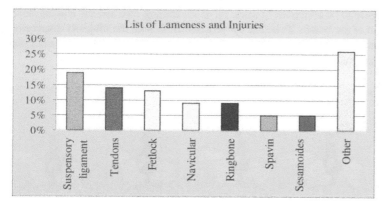

Fig.7-6: British Army: types of lameness listing, as compiled from the Regimental Veterinary Officer's fitness register (Ivon Bell, 1994).

Lameness patterns were also looked at (Fig.7-6). The most common type of injury documented was associated with the suspensory ligament, which accounted for 26% of all lameness, and of those, the left fore was the most affected (Fig.7-7). Comparison of the two hind limbs illustrated the right hind was the most subjected to injury, concluding that the left diagonal was the diagonal most likely to exhibit an unlevel action in trot.

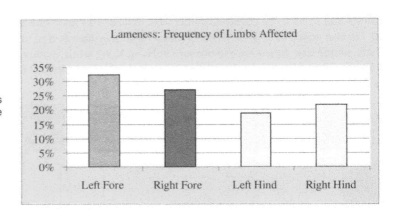

Fig.7-7: British Army: frequency of limbs affected by lameness, as compiled from the Shoeing Roll Army Book (Ivon Bell, 1994).

Fig. 7-8: The Rising Trot (left diagonal); some animals show a preference for one diagonal.

In the rising trot the rider sits in the saddle as one diagonal pair of hooves contact the ground, then rises out of the saddle as the other diagonal pair of hooves contact the ground.

The diagonal pair of limbs upon which the rider sits is named after the forelimb, in this illustration the rider is sitting on the left diagonal.

It is generally accepted that when schooling, the diagonal upon which the rider sits comprises the outside forelimb and the inside hindlimb.

When riding on the road, the centre of the road becomes as the centre of the schooling arena, with the rider using their inside leg to push the horse's hindquarters toward the kerb side and away from the centre of the road. The rider's inside leg is also supported by the use of both the outside and inside rein; this effectively bends the horse, keeping the hindquarters safely away from traffic while allowing the horse to see any vehicles approaching. With the horse bent in such a manner, it is customary then to sit on the outside fore, inside hind, diagonal.

To date it is not clear how the rules of the road will affect the symmetry of the horse and the wear of the shoes but the advice given to any rider is, be aware and change diagonals from time to time.

Shoe wear was something that was also examined throughout Sergeant Bell's detailed study. The wearing of the front shoe towards the outside of the toe was common ('breakover') and the uneven wearing of the lateral branch of the hind shoes was something that was also noted. Trials were carried out with horses at the trot; aluminium hind shoes were fitted prior to a work period of 2-4 hours. It was thought the camber of the road increased the wear to the lateral branch of the right shoe but no apparent wear difference could be properly identified when the animal was asked to work on its 'preferred diagonal'.

The term preferred or favoured diagonal, which the horse may 'throw' a rider on to, is not something which has been scientifically defined, instead it is an action which in itself may be quite subjective, being based upon how comfortable or how 'at one' the horse and rider may feel. However, the preferred diagonal suggested by owners and riders, would seem to be consistently made up of the trailing fore and the leading hind. So of the horses looked at by Sergeant Bell, with the majority displaying larger right hooves, we would expect them to prefer the left diagonal, the diagonal which was shown as the most likely to be unlevel.

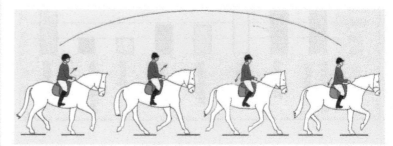

Fig.7-8: The Rising Trot (left diagonal).

PREFERRED OR DOMINANT DIAGONAL

Why should the left diagonal be found to be the most unlevel? The answer is simple; more lameness occurs in the left fore/right hind diagonal because it just so happens to be the diagonal which is the most inherently preferred. This readiness of the equine to have such a definite way of moving is now a fact, which is fortunately something that is fast becoming readily understood. So much so, that many practitioners now feel more willing to accept that most lameness problems are as a result of a cycle of repeated trauma rather than being from one single event. To understand how this occurs, we only need to look to the world of sport. Think of rugby players and boxers having cauliflower ears, roadrunners having bad knees and tennis players having tennis elbow. Repetitive strain injuries are even a constant source of problems to farriers themselves, with most farriers at some time or another suffering from a bad back.

The recognition of asymmetry and establishing or predicting which limbs may be the most prone to injury could, if known, influence stable management routines and training programs. This essential knowledge could even be used to help owners decide which of their horses are the most likely to achieve a desired goal in any particular chosen discipline.

The questions of what is acceptable asymmetry and why horses go lame in one leg are the questions which have driven the research and the line of inquiry of at least two well-known authorities, Dr Deb Bennett and Tony Gonzales. Both have devoted considerable amounts of time in finding their answers to those questions, each writing books upon asymmetry, while others like Ernie Gray, a distinguished American farrier, have taken it upon themselves to discover the fundamental origin of the cause of asymmetry.

The idea that asymmetry is the result of some naturally inherent preferred behaviour pattern is a question which has exercised the minds of many. The suggested causes are limb dominance, eye dominance, respiratory/locomotor coupling (a pattern of breathing linked to motion, see Fig.7-9), diagonal orientation and brain lateralization, with each factor thought to play its role in the formation of any natural asymmetry within the equine. Whatever the cause, its existence is to be found to a greater or lesser degree in each and every horse with the defining line between a naturally occurring unlevel action and lameness becoming ever less distinct.

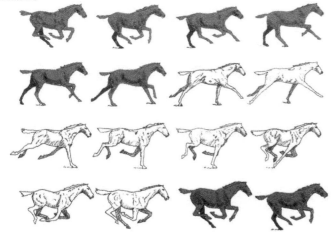

Fig 7-9: Respiratory/locomotor coupling:(after Cook, W. R., 1992, & Hayes, H. M., 1893).

Fig 7-9: An illustration based upon an idea by Bob Cook; one spring morning, in 1963, as Bob cantered a client's horse to test its wind, he suddenly had a 'eureka' moment. For as he rode he became aware that the motion of the horse was engendered by the synchronised rhythm of hoof beat and breath; the horse was breathing in time with its legs.

As he researched his discovery, through what literature he could find, his euphoria became short lived, as he soon realised that a Dr Wittke, in Germany, had made the very same observations; these observations were later to become known as 'respiratory/locomotor coupling'.

In the illustration, inspiration takes place when the hind legs are weight bearing (black horses), and expiration takes place when the forelegs are weight bearing (white horses)

Asymmetry, handedness and limb dominance has exercised the minds of many; with the causes and explanations thought to be many and various, with each factor considered to play its role within the holistic make-up of the horse. It would seem illogical not to link naturally inherent preferred behaviour with every aspect of being associated with movement and stance; respiratory/locomotor coupling is just one such aspect.

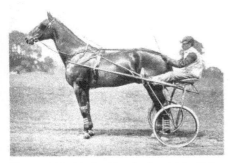

Fig. 7-10: The Racing Standardbred, taken from Axe, J .W., 1905.

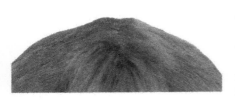

Fig. 7-11: Tuber sacrale ('hunter's bump').

Photograph showing an old horse with 'hunter's bumps' and a slightly increased muscle development on the left hind.

HINDLIMB ASYMMETRY

The world of Standardbred racing has attracted considerable research. Standardbreds (Fig.7-10) are so called because of their lineage, having been selected only through their ability to either trot or pace a measured mile within a standard fixed time. Racing Standardbreds are divided into two groups; there are those with the natural ability to pace (this is where the lateral pairs of limbs move together) and those, which naturally trot (the trot is a symmetrical gait where the diagonally opposite pair of limbs move together). According to researchers, G. Dalin and S. Drevemo, whose work has focussed upon hindquarter asymmetry in Standardbred trotters, asymmetry can be considered to lead to a poor performance. This assumption was reflected by a reduced percentage of winnings of one of the study groups examined. Asymmetry within the body shape of any equine can be difficult to define, calling upon experienced and impartial judgements. In fact, within that particular study group, comprising 500 horses, no marked asymmetry was to be found in 92%, a total forming 6% of those studied were noted as having a higher left tuber sacrale than the right, with only 2% exhibiting a higher right tuber sacrale (Fig.7-11).

So why should the left tuber sacrale be higher than the right? Well, it is possible that this is yet another pattern which may also be attributed to both habits of stance and movement. Another recurrent observation, which has been noted by a wide variety of equestrian authors writing about asymmetry, has been the overall suggestion that more muscle bulk can be readily identified in a slightly higher proportion of left hind limbs. These two observations may be linked and explained when a closer look at the way the crooked horse moves is considered. The hindquarters comprise a group of large muscles overlying and enveloping the pelvic region making it difficult to see or feel the skeletal framework. As a result, where the tuber sacrale appear asymmetrical it is likely that this observation is due to a larger development of muscle on one side, rather than through any misalignment of the sacroiliac joint. This pronounced muscle development is thought to be due to the range of weight-bearing motion produced by the preferred trailing hind, while the preferred leading limb, it has been suggested, can be sometimes identified by a more developed gaskin, just like a right-footed person, who may have a more developed right calf. The reason for that is that the muscles in both the forearm and gaskin are in constant use both in motion and during the act of grazing and so the one-sided animal may have a greater development of those muscles, particularly on one side, the dominant side.

In another study looking at asymmetry in trotters, a group of 8-month-old Standardbreds was assessed prior to any training given. Many of these animals were found to show notable left-right asymmetries of movement and this was thought to be strong evidence in favour of an inherent laterality or handedness when asymmetries were found in animals so young. This suggestion was further supported by the fact that after these same animals had undergone race training;

they were re-evaluated at the age of 18 months. This new assessment proved somewhat interesting, as it was to highlight that those differences between the left and right sides, which had previously been observed, had now become even more pronounced. Therefore, a conclusion which may be drawn from these observations, is that because these animals were asked to trot regularly and as fast as possible, it is likely that the asymmetries, which could well be attributed to those equines having a preferred diagonal, were encouraged. The question is then raised that if asymmetries are recognised and appropriate work regimes undertaken, could the equine's working life be improved?

THE CROOKED HORSE

So what can this wealth of evidence mean to the owner, the farrier and the vet; and how will our new improved understanding affect the way in which we manage the horse? Simply by being aware of the probability that asymmetry will exist to some degree in each and every horse will in itself bring with it a new found perception. In fact, that which has been in the past considered abnormal may now be viewed as being quite normal with asymmetry being a product of the horse's own natural balance.

What form of asymmetry is the owner most likely to see? A great many owners will be quite aware that their horse has got odd feet and a few of those will also notice a difference in their equine's shoulder bulk but most will notice that their horse will go much better on one rein than another.

Ideally, horses should move straight with each hind leg following in the same track as the foreleg on the same side, each limb sharing equally the same weight bearing functions as the corresponding limb on the opposite side; however, with the crooked horse this is not so.

The crooked horse is so called because of the way that it moves; in dogs, the type of movement is often referred to as crabbing or side winding. The term is derived from the way a sea-crab crawls forwards in a sidewise action with the animal moving, during the act of progression, with its body turned at an angle to its forward line of travel. In dogs, when this action is duplicated, the dog may be said to be moving in three tracks, this is where, in theory, the paw-prints seem to lie in three parallel lines. Likewise, in horses when this type of action is replicated the animal is also said to move in three tracks (Fig.7-12).

The crooked horse is a horse which prefers its own habitual way of going, leading with its limbs on one side and trailing with the limbs on the other (canter). It also has a tendency to trot on a preferred diagonal, usually comprising the preferred trailing fore and leading hind, which can be identified during both the canter and the gallop. In doing so, the limbs within each pair (front and hind) do not perform the same tasks or ranges of movement. In the canter and the gallop, the trailing hind reaches forward but not as far as the leading hind; it

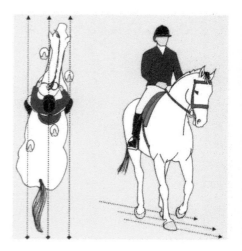

Fig.7-12: An illustration showing the horse, in trot, moving in three tracks.

When a horse moves straight, it is said to move in two tracks.

In trot, a crooked horse will move in three: the outside hind in one, the dominant hind and the diagonal fore in another and the dominant fore on the inside track. The head may very well tilt to allow the dominant eye better vision, thereby turning the head toward the less dextrous side. In canter, however, this same horse will exhibit a natural tendency to straighten up.

contacts with the ground earlier but provides a greater thrust. The leading hind then lands but reaches much further forward producing a pelvic twist, which causes the hindquarters to move at an angle to the chosen line of progression. It is this twisting which then produces the effect where the horse is said to move in three tracks and it is this action, which has been likened to the dressage movement 'haunches in'. During this action, the horse may place the trailing hind in one track, the trailing fore and dominant hind in a central track and the lead fore in the inside track. This asymmetric style of movement, if habitually recreated, produces a greater muscle development on the preferred trailing hind and a noticeable development of muscle on the shoulder of the leading fore. This style of movement is also thought to affect the muscle development of the leading or dominant hind creating a larger gaskin. This is because during its cycle of movement, it produces a lateral swing similar to the dressage movement known as 'leg yielding' and in doing so is placed more centrally under the trunk of the horse close to the animal's centre of gravity.

The crooked horse comes in a variety of packages but this outline described is without doubt the most common, with the right side being the most dominant and the majority of horses preferring to trot on the left diagonal. So if the owner knows their horse has preferences in trot and canter and exhibits a definite grazing pattern what can they do?

THE OWNER / RIDER INFLUENCE

Owners and riders are often blamed for creating their crooked horse with the suggestion that their equine's crookedness is somehow related to their handling or riding. This can be true to some extent, the main failing of most horse owners lies within their own inability to recognise just how asymmetric their equines are. If they did, it is possible they could then do something to help rectify their horse's unevenness and ultimately, in turn, help their horse to remain sound.

Dressage is an equestrian sport with origins dating back to the ancient Greeks, who established its basic principles. It was born out of the need to improve and maintain a high level of masterly horsemanship. An army's cavalry was for centuries one of its most battle-winning assets and supremacy in the field was so often decided upon by the ability of its mounted troops to either wield or fire weapons while continuing to maintain a decisive command of the horses they were astride. Today it is a disciplined stylised form of competition riding practised to display a high level of horsemastership.

In effect, the essence of dressage is about utilising and developing the equine's natural movements through dedicated training, working to perfect these natural acts of progression so that they may be faultlessly executed upon command, which requires an overall fitness and a natural dexterity of the horse. The rider can then develop the equine's suppleness, which is needed to produce the high level of controlled balance required for competition.

Unfortunately, the crooked horse, in its extreme, has little hope of proving to be a top dressage horse. This is because despite the fact that the way in which it has a natural tendency to move may replicate some of the exercises required for this discipline, it may prove extremely difficult for the rider to get the horse to mirror those moves. Dressage at whatever level has a habit of discovering just how crooked any horse may be and this is little wonder; after all, the word dressage is derived from the French verb 'dresser', which means to train, to adjust and to straighten-out. An active, organised schooling regime is exactly what is required if these animals are to be helped. All horses can be improved with benefits not only to their overall health, fitness and dexterity but also through this process, an enhanced level of mutual appreciation will be achieved between both horse and rider. After all, this was and essentially still is the reasoning behind dressage; to bring both horse and rider together into a higher level of understanding and to help them both last longer.

THE FARRIERY INFLUENCE

The crooked horse is the horse that effectively does not move straight, and because the horse does not move straight, its hooves are unlikely to be either the same size or shape. Its shoe wear may not be even, with one hind shoe wearing out far more rapidly on one side. Shoe loss may also be a problem with the smaller of the front hooves belonging to the apparently longer distal limb. This creates a greater risk of that shoe being torn off at the beginning of any shoeing cycle; however, the shoe on the larger foot has a propensity to sink inside the hoof, becoming loose near the end of the shoeing cycle.

The farrier is often faced with the unenviable task of being the one who is expected to create a horse with two evenly matched pairs of hooves. However, although it is the farrier who is the one given the role of levelling the hooves it is beyond the powers of any farrier to level the horse; that unlevel action cannot be fixed simply by the farrier alone. The task is really down to the owner and rider but the initial step they need to make and be reminded of, is for them to recognise that they have a crooked horse, so that they themselves can take the appropriate action.

What the farrier has to do is tackle the effects of the crooked horse. An upright hoof will need to be trimmed and lowered at the heels, redressing the balance, and a flat hoof will need to be shod with enough length at the heels to provide the support required. Occasionally, added support can be provided for a flat hoof, by the use of an egg-bar shoe, which, at times, may prove to be very useful. The upright fore-hoof may also require special attention because of shoe loss. Here traditional style pencilled heels may help to reduce the risk of the shoe being struck off; failing that, overreach boots may also prove a useful suggestion. It is worthwhile remembering that shoe loss has a tendency to occur either out in the field or when the horse is out of control; shoes never just simply fall off.

TAKE HOME MESSAGE

The crooked horse, or in fact every horse, requires the mutual understanding of both horse owner and farrier; with the owner appreciating that good farriery effectively deals with symptoms and not causes and with the farrier acknowledging that his or her input, no matter how important, does have its limitations.

Crooked riders and inept farriers do not create crooked horses. However, corrective schooling and good farriery, when practised as part of an organised response, can produce both the conditioning and the foundations essential to bring about the necessary environment needed to straighten those horses out.

Good farriery is important at all times, and it is by means of their continued daily practices that farriers get to see hooves on a very regular basis. It is through their very unique role that farriers are, in fact, the ones best placed to recognise and monitor any hoof changes. The hoof is plastic by its nature and as such is subject to any force which is placed upon it; force changes its form (hoof deformation) but unlike tissue, which is elastic, it does not readily return to its original shape. One of the effects of handedness or crookedness is hoof deformation, but thoughtful management by the owner, minimising grazing times, bearing the welfare of the horse in mind and placing forage and water off the ground and using rubber matting inside the stable, can help reduce this effect. Then, with the farrier periodically returning to redress the hoof, he will be able to discuss with the owner the success of any management and work routines. Communication and teamwork are after all, pre-requisites of good farriery

THE CROOKED HORSE: SUMMARY

1. Many horses exhibit behavioural patterns, which influence hoof shape, the most obvious one being the act of grazing. Through the prolonged act of grazing, 'one-sided' animals develop differing hoof shapes.

2. The 'grazing stance' is a good indicator of the preferred lead.

3. The 'grazing stance' reflects the leading-limb ~ trailing-limb configuration. The flatter hoof being associated with the leading limb and the more up-right hoof being associated with the trailing limb.

4. During the canter, in all horses, the leading legs are on the same side; the leading limbs are so called because they stride out further.

5. The dominant hind and non-dominant fore will invariably be the animals preferred diagonal in trot.

6. In the trot, the rider sits on the dominant hind and rises on the dominant fore.

7. The horse will bend more easily to the dominant side (hollow side).

8. As the horse moves it may be perceived as moving in three tracks, rather like the dressage movement 'shoulder in'. During this action, the horse may place the trailing hind in one track, the trailing fore and dominant hind in a central track and the lead fore in the inside track.

9. When the horse moves in this fashion the dominant hind may be subject to an exaggerated lateral swing, as it places it hoof underneath its body.

10. In canter, the leading limbs land at an acute angle; the trailing limbs land at an obtuse angle. Combined with the habits of stance, these actions will create apparent leg-length differences.

11. Trailing forelimbs have an apparent longer distal limb, while leading forelimbs will have an apparently shorter distal limb. This disparity will encourage the animal to bend towards the hollow side.

12. The limb-length disparity will also increase the risk of shoe loss on the smaller hoof of the non-dominant fore (trailing-limb). This is because limb-length and hoof shape will affect the stride length.

13. The results of the horse's asymmetric behaviour will result in an undesirable functional asymmetry ('crookedness').

14. Physical asymmetry will also be apparent in any number of ways, hoof size and shape, disparity in the shoulders, lower chest and hindquarters, all of which are indicative of the 'crooked' horse.

15. Finally, uneven shoe wear is likely, particularly on the lateral side of the dominant hind.

BIBLIOGRAPHY

'If you take ideas from one source it's called plagiarism. When you take ideas from five its called research'

Back, W., Clayton, H. M., *Equine Locomotion* (Harcourt Publishers Ltd 2001)

Batchelor, D.C., *'Short Leg Syndrome'* http://www.chiroweb.com/archives/20/18/02.html (Access March 2007)

Bell, I., 'Evaluating the Shoeing and Associated Hoof problems of Household Cavalry Horses' (*4ᵗʰ International Farriery and Lameness Seminar Handbook* 1994)

Bennett, D., 'Lessons from Woody' & 'True Collection', *ESI Knowledge Base.* http://www.equinestudies.org/knowledge_base/woody.html (Access March 2007)

Coren, S., *Left Hander* (The Free Press, 1993)

Clayton, H., McPhail Chair Presentations http://www.cvm.msu.edu/dressage/articles/index.htm (Access March 2007)

Deuel, N. R., Lawrence, L. M., 'Laterality in the gallop gait of horses', *Journal of Biomechanics,* volume 20, No. 6 p. 645-649, 1987.

Elliott, R. P., *The New Dogsteps* (Howell Book House, 1983)

Gonzales, A. Z., *Proper Balance Movement: A diary of lameness* (REF Publishing, 1986)

Gonzales, A. Z., *Proper Balance Movement: Part 1, Confirmation & Lamenesses, video* (Lawlor Productions 1992)

Grandage, J., *Horses in Motion*, 32 min video (Australian Equine Research Foundation) © University of Queensland, Australia

Gray, E., *'Equine Asymmetrical Dexterity or, The Preferred Lead Syndrome'*, The Farrier & Hoofcare Resource Center (www.horseshoes.com) Access March 2007

Harris, S. H., *Horse Gaits Balance and Movement* (Macmillan Publishing Co. 1993)

Hayes, M. H., *Points of the Horse* (Arco Publishing Company, Inc., 1976)

MacLeod, D., *The Rules of Work: A Practical Engineering Guide to Ergonomics* (Taylor & Francis © 2000)

Morris, S., *Straightness* http://www.classicaldressage.co.uk (Access March 2007)

Muybridge, E., *Animals in Motion* (Dover Publications, Inc., 1957)

Rossdale, P.D., Greet, T.R.C., Harris, P.A., Green, R.E., Hall, S., *et al.*, *Guardians of the Horse: Past Present and Future* (British Equine Veterinary Association and Romney Publications, 1999)

Smythe, R. H., Goody, P. H., *Horse Structure and Movement* (J. A. Allen, London, 1993)

Stashak, T. S., *Adams' Lameness in Horses* (Lea & Febiger, 4ᵗʰ edition 1987)

Turner, T. A., Equine Podiatry (Northern Virginia Equine) http://www.equipodiatry.com/hoofbal.htm (Access March 2007)

Unequal Leg Length: The leg is too long (usually). http://www.totaljoints.info/Long_leg_TH.htm (Access March 2007)

8: Farriery in practice

REASONS FOR FARRIERY

The fundamental reason that we shoe our horses is to improve their well-being and usefulness. Each hoof is in a continuous state of change through deformation, growth and wear and to counteract these actions, we call upon the skill of the farrier to redress the hoof's balance with the aim of creating a conditional equilibrium. The farrier achieves this through the act of trimming, or trimming and the application of a shoe: these are the actions commonly known as farriery.

DEFORMATION AND GROWTH: THE NEED TO REDRESS THE HOOF'S BALANCE

Suspended within the hoof capsule, the pedal bone is supported by its natural covering (Fig.8-1). The hoof capsule should reflect the bone's shape, the angle at which it lies and the direction in which it is facing. However this spatial positioning is not fixed, instead it is a compliant arrangement influenced by a constant succession of change.

Displacement and adaptation create the balance of the hoof as multidimensional loading, growth and, wear continuously modify its form.

Our familiarity with the horse's hoof belies its complexity; the hoof has a natural design and makeup that serves as both the foundation for the limb and as a compensatory device. This composite structure acts to dampen concussion and disperse energy. It is able to multitask because of the qualities of the materials from which it is constructed.

The hoof is engineered from specialised horn sharing uniquely differing properties having been bound or laminated together to provide both strength and pliability. Collectively this union of tissue is able to sustain great loads, absorbing impact, resisting stress and accommodating wear. As an assembly, we refer to this structure as the hoof capsule and as a unit; its mass could be described as possessing a viscoelastic form.

The viscoelastic properties of the hoof capsule make it capable of withstanding sudden impact. It does this through deforming; absorbing energy as the hoof strikes the ground but then, as the hoof is lifted off

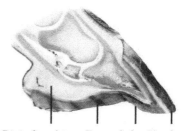

Digital cushion...Frog...Sole...Hoof wall

Fig. 8-1: The hoof capsule (Photo supplied by Samuel Beeley, farrier, UK).

The pedal bone is suspended within its natural covering.

The hoof is a composite structure formed by various tissues bonded together to create the form we are familiar with: the hoof capsule.

The tissues that form the hoof are of a viscoelastic nature.

When the hoof is loaded briefly, the hoof's shape deforms but quickly returns, as the hoof is unloaded. However, if the load is applied for a long period, a plastic deformation will occur and the hoof's shape will change.

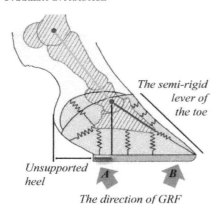

The semi-rigid lever of the toe

Unsupported heel

A   B

The direction of GRF at (A)impact and (B) break-over

Fig. 8-2: The spatial arrangement of the pedal bone within the hoof capsule is subject to change through deformation, growth and wear.

Regardless of whether the hoof is shod or unshod, if the ground contact area is too far forward the hoof will become inherently unstable. This will place the palmar structures, at the back of the hoof, under load.

Long, over grown hooves are liable to deform, as they extend the amount of unsupported heel and increase the strain on semi-rigid lever of the toe.

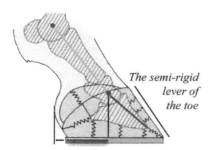

The semi-rigid lever of the toe

The ground contact area at the heel supports the reinforcement/coupling at the back of the hoof

Fig. 8-3: Understanding what the hoof should look like is a 'must do'.

Flat hooves receive a greater load at the heels, while more upright hooves receive a greater load to the toe.

the ground, it releases that energy, elastically returning to its original shape. This has prompted other authors to describe the viscoelastic tissues of the hoof as sharing a similar type of quality to that of 'memory foam'. However when a load is applied gradually over a longer period a 'creep effect' can occur. If a material, or in this case the hoof, is loaded with a constant stress which is maintained or repeated over a sufficiently long time, then fatigue sets in and the material or structure can fail. This results in a plastic deformation, affecting both the function and the properties of the tissues involved. Ridges characterise hoof deformation as the horn tubules buckle under their load and these are the telltale signs that the hoof capsule has changed its shape.

Creep or hoof deformation is a very real effect that should not be trivialised, as it can and does have a considerable bearing upon the biomechanics of the limb. It is because of this that rebalancing the hoof forms such a quintessential aspect of farriery: the shape of the hoof having such a great influence on both impact and loading.

For horses that go barefoot, this phenomenon does not provide a huge challenge but it does provide the main reason for trimming. However, for those horses that are shod, for the farriers that apply the shoes and for the owners that are responsible for the welfare of those horses, deformation is a very real problem that needs constant managing. So regardless of whether the horse is shod or unshod, all hooves will require some sort of monitoring if they are to remain pain free.

Shoes that are too short, or shoes which have been left on too long, will leave the back of the hoof effectively under a constant load, making this issue an ever-present area of concern. Similarly, unshod hooves that have heels which have a ground surface contact area positioned too far forward will also require regular monitoring. So a familiarisation of how the hoof should look is a 'must do'.

Deformation is a phenomenon that can occur to any section of the hoof wall but it is the front half of the hoof, the shape and length of the toe, that most observers will notice first. The effects can be quite conspicuous with the hoof wall frequently taking on a concave appearance, punctuated by converging ridges and a substantial lengthening of the toe. Long toes are the associated by-product of reduced heel height, commonly known as collapsed heels, with the hoof's exterior being a good indicator of the angle of the pedal bone. Upright heels are also indicative of the pedal bones spatial location, with the steep angle of the toe reflecting in the angle at which the bone is positioned; again, like the flatter hooves, the wall may also take on a concave form.

The hoof's shape and angle is a good predictor of limb loading both for when the horse is at rest or moving. Horses that display hooves that are seemingly different in size and shape, will have acquired their dissimilarities through the different loading patterns applied to those hooves, low-heeled hooves being exposed to a greater load at the heel and upright heels being subjected to a greater load at the toe. The back portion of the hoof is the part of the hoof that is responsible for providing the necessary input to support the weight of the horse and the toe of the hoof being the portion that acts as an output to provide propulsion during locomotion. During the final moments of progression, the horn at the toe is pushed into the ground surface, which responds with an equal but opposite force driven against the horn. This predictable but necessary sequence not only provides the effect for a final push off before the hoof is flicked back but it also inevitably places added strain on the semi-rigid lever formed by the hoof at the toe. This action not only causes the horn tubules to buckle under the load, it also creates the abradant wear pattern known as breakover.

While deformation reduces some aspects of the hoof, the opposing features may continue to increase their length or height through an unrestricted growth. Therefore, reduced heels accompany long toes and restricted growth at the toe will accompany an increase in heel height. These seemingly sometimes minor shape changes, then impact on the biomechanics of the limb, affecting both impact and loading patterns. Therefore, excess growth needs to be removed and deformation addressed because the hoof's shape and its relationship with the skeletal limb is, without doubt, the indispensable affiliation that is the key to soundness.

SHOE WEAR

Shoe wear takes place wherever there is movement. As the shoe contacts the ground during progression, a certain amount of sliding will take place. The amount of sliding is dependent on a number of factors including the type and manufacture of the shoe and the ground conditions. Studies have been carried out by farriers and veterinarians in an attempt to record and determine how much slide is essential during the process of deceleration as the hoof contacts the ground during progression and how much, as well as how little, slippage can induce excessive strain and concussion. Nevertheless, slippage is a normal occurrence and during this slippage, friction takes place and wherever there is friction there is wear.

Movement takes place between the heels of the shoe and the ground surface upon initial contact and then over the entire ground surface of the shoe until the hoof becomes stationary, although it should be acknowledged that any point of zero motion has to be considered as theoretical. However, on both the fore and hind shoes it is relatively normal for one side of the shoe to wear more than the other. This is usually due to the repositioning of the hoof during the stance phase as the joints within the limb, which are hinge joints, travel through their own peculiar range of motion. This type of joint is created with the upper and lower bones taking in a different plane of motion, so for example, as the stifle moves outwards, the hock twists in, likewise as the stifle moves inwards (during the stance phase) then the hock twists out. This action causes the shoe to wear as the hoof repositions itself, skewing around and twisting while the foot is both weight-bearing and in contact with the ground (Figs. 8-4).

Shoe wear also takes place at the toe of the fore-hooves and this is commonly identified as the breakover. The action known as breakover begins as the heels are levered off the ground. In that same instant, the toe of the hoof becomes a fulcrum and a frictional wear takes place as the

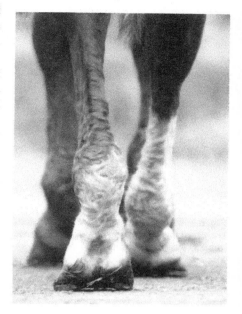

Figs. 8-4: Here the right hind can be seen to reposition itself during the stance phase; this will cause wear to the lateral branch of the shoe (Photo: J. Watts).

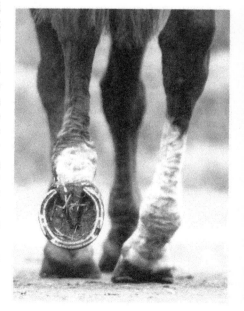

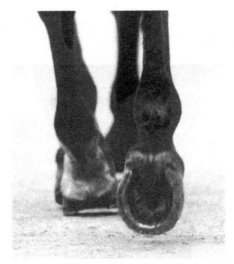

Fig. 8-5: More wear can be seen on the lateral branch of this right hind shoe but as it travels through the swing phase, the hoof at the toe also catches the ground surface (Photo: J. Watts).

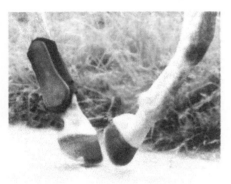

Fig. 8-6: Hooves move so closely to one another that a misstep can cause them to interfere, which may result in a lost shoe.

hoof pushes against the ground surface. The wear pattern frequently observed tends to reflect the direction of the knee relative to the direction of the foot and so acts as a good indicator of the geometry of the limb. This wear pattern almost invariably occurs to the lateral aspect of the shoe and this should be considered normal. Shoeing plans directed at attempting to change the breakover are not recommended, as they are likely to create torsional forces within the limb.

Hind shoes can also be affected by wear at the toe. During the swing phase after breakover, some horses, because of their action, catch or scrape the toe of the hind shoe on the ground as it travels forward (Fig. 8-5). This can also happen with front hooves, although it is more unusual and when it does occur, the horse is likely to stumble.

The wear of the shoe can determine when the horse requires shoeing. If the shoe is too worn, it can increase the hoof's slide times and so increase the risk of injury due to excessive slippage. Shoes as they become thinner can also lead to loose and lost shoes.

LOST SHOES

Lost shoes are another reason to re-shoe. Those shoes that are lost during the first half of the shoeing cycle are generally the result of some unpremeditated movement due to either the horse being uncollected and out of control while being ridden, or because they have been out in the field in uneven and slippery conditions. All horses can lose shoes but those horses that tend to lose shoes more regularly than others tend also to be those which lose one particular shoe more than any other. Recurrent shoe loss of one particular shoe happens to be both indicative and an effect of asymmetric horses; these horses can test both farriers and owners alike. Farriers need to balance feet, owners need to balance their horse; schooling, management and over-reach boots are all applications which need to be considered by the owner.

Horses can often be seen out of control charging and galloping around the field and at those times, it seems little wonder that shoes are lost. Shoes never simply 'drop off' they are pulled off. Worn, smooth shoes are often lost because they give little traction, making the horse's footing less secure and liable to uncontrolled movements. This increases the chance of one hoof catching the shoe on another hoof. In addition, the diminished strength of worn shoes means there will be less material within the body of the nail head to hold the shoe in place. Horseshoes are secured to the hoof by nails that are shaped to countersink into the main body of the shoe. When the heads are worn down, there is less to hold the shoe on tightly.

WHEN TO CALL THE FARRIER

Being aware of when and why the horse needs shoeing is the first essential step in understanding farriery because that helps to determine when to call upon the farrier.

Many people make this decision by gauging the shoeing intervals. Those who do this, often tend to have their horses looked at every 6-8 weeks. This planning makes life easier both for the owner and the farrier and regularly shod horses are generally better behaved. Contacting the farrier and giving at least a week's notice is ideal although not always possible. Lost shoes and unsound horses may require attention that is more urgent and farriers should endeavour to have their business organised to allow them to deal with such events.

The reasons for using a particular farrier may be many and varied. Accessibility has to be high on the list as a farrier who is based many miles away will have to allow, and charge for, travelling time if they are to come to the horse. Alternatively, the horse will need to be taken to the farrier, which is not always convenient. Local farriers need to be supported and encouraged; it makes good all-round sense.

When contacting the farrier it may be useful to tell him the type, height of animal and the kind of work the horse usually does. Even more helpful would be to say if you thought the animal's feet were large or small relative to its height and weight, better still measuring the hoof or the old shoes can also be a help. To do this you will need a ruler to measure across the widest part of the hoof (Fig. 8-7) and then from where the outer edge of the toe to where the heels of the shoe should end (Fig. 8-8). These two measurements should give the farrier a good idea about what size shoes to bring.

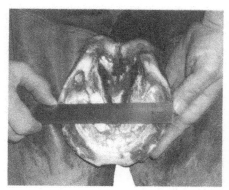
Fig. 8-7: Measuring the width of the hoof (Photo: Alex Gill).

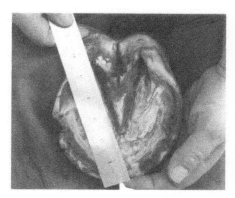
Fig. 8-8: Measuring the distance from the toe to where the heels of a new shoe will end (Photo: Alex Gill).

PREPARING FOR THE FARRIER

The better the facilities that you have for the farrier to carry out his or her task the higher and more consistent the standards of work you can expect. To ask someone to shoe a horse without assistance in the rain or blazing sunshine with the horse simply tied up to a fence post without thought to the safety and well-being of either farrier or horse is both unacceptable and Dickensian. Not unreasonably, any farrier will want to work in an area protected from the elements, so providing a good clean stable or shoeing area is essential. Forward planning will always pay dividends beginning with the decision of where to site your stable and its design. Vehicular access is very important, as carrying heavy equipment over muddy fields is far from ideal (Fig. 8-9). Good windows and lights are a must-have. It is essential that the farrier can see what he is doing and it's important to remember too that when horses are held or tied, they tend to dislike facing into the dark. A clean, dry, well-lit area, with a good floor surface is ideal but the main criterion has to be an area where the horse is at its most manageable, and at ease with its surroundings (Fig. 8-10). In busy yards, horses because of their nature can become restless if other horses are led in or out of the area, or if other horses are being fed; so scheduling and finding the best time slot for the horse to be shod is very important. Horses are creatures of habit; they do not like it when they are taken out of their daily routine and they certainly do not like it when they think everyone else is being fed but them! Thought and planning are needed at all times if shoeing is to be carried out in safety; no running or

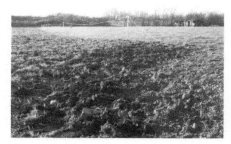
Fig. 8-9: Vehicular access to the shoeing area is essential; carrying heavy tools across muddy fields should be unnecessary.

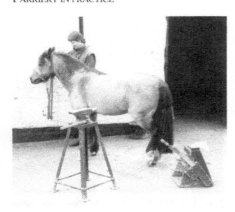

Fig. 8-10: Clean animals, in a good environment and managed by a responsible handler, will help ease the task

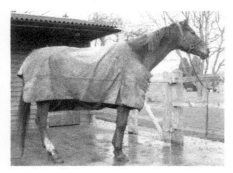

Fig. 8-11: If the horse has a dirty rug on, remove it.

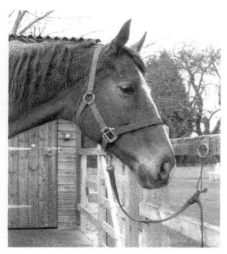

Fig. 8-12: Having the horse tied to a breakable linkage is an important safety feature; here string is used.

sudden movements should be made by anyone either attending to the horse or within the shoeing area.

Clean legs and hooves free from mud or wet is another help for the farrier. Mud and wet affect the ability of the farrier to carry out the necessary tasks, as the tools can become slippery to handle and rasps can become clogged. If the horse is wearing either a dirty rug or one which impairs the horse's free movement, remove it (Fig. 8-11). The farrier's job is bound to be difficult and dirty anyway so try wherever possible to make it a little less so. The more satisfied the farrier is with the horse, the conditions and the owner, the more able he is to work well.

The owner also needs to decide whether the animal is to be tied up or managed by a competent handler. Whichever is considered the best option, the farrier will still require assistance and supervision. Well-behaved horses are generally fine if tied up, particularly if given a hay-net to keep them occupied.

When tying up the horse, always ensure for maximum safety, that a breakable linkage is in use between the lead rope and the object to which it is tied (Fig. 8-12). This is because if the horse were to pull back and fight against its restraint the situation could easily become dangerous. However, once the linkage is broken the affray is usually ended and the animal will soon become calmer.

HOLDING THE HORSE

Next, in the interests of safety the horse needs to be well handled. It is not within the farrier's remit to train and break horses; that is the responsibility of the owner..

Holding horses is a much-underrated skill; ask any vet or farrier. Some farriers and vets even prefer to employ their own assistants. Unfortunately, although there are many owners able to hold the end of a rope, few can competently hold a horse. There are those who think they can control a horse while using their mobile phone, drink coffee, even sit down and generally relax. The boredom factor of the job for these people can be so overwhelming, that when the horse suddenly does move they then have a tendency to overreact. Horsemanship is not a prerequisite of owning a horse but then neither is it for a farrier whose training focuses upon the acquisition of the hand skills required to do the job and to understand the theory behind those practices rather than horse-handling skills.

Horsemanship is a combination of learned skills and natural instincts. It is not something that people are going to pick up just from reading books, watching videos or going on weekend courses although all these things help. It is something that is acquired through time and the application of common sense; so Mums and Dads, leaving your eight-year-old daughter on her own to hold the horse for the farrier is just a recipe for disaster! It really helps for the handler to know and understand horses well enough to anticipate what could happen and prevent it from happening before it does.

Horses can often take their lead from their handlers. A calm positive approach can be reassuring both to the horse and to the farrier. After all, the farrier's safety is reliant upon whoever is managing the horse. Knowing how to behave while the horse is shod and knowing what the farrier expects of the handler is a very important aspect of farriery. The handler should at all times stand on the same side as the farrier, facing the horse, so that they can see exactly what is going on (Fig. 8-13). The only time the handler should stand on the other side of the horse's head is when the farrier takes a front foot forward for rasping (Fig. 8-14). In this position, the handler will be able to keep the horse's head in line with its centre of mass. If the horse has its head to one side or is allowed to stretch its neck out, the centre of mass shifts and it just makes the job a whole lot harder for the farrier, who has to struggle with the weight of the horse.

Some horses find shoeing a bit tedious and so occupying them with the distraction of feed can be really quite useful: here again the hay-net can prove to be very effective as a pacifier (Fig. 8-15). Limited hard feed also has its uses as do carrots but these should be used sparingly when the farrier is nailing the shoe on. Horsemanship is about being aware and feeding can sometimes have a negative affect on the horse's behaviour because some horses simply get grumpy and impatient when food is around.

There is a lot to remember and think about when holding the horse for the farrier but the main thing is to pay attention at all times and keep in control. Do not let the horse nibble or lick the farrier, horses can all bite. Keep the horse in one spot; don't let it wander about. Constantly moving a heavy tool box either out of the way or back to where the horse is now standing can be very tiresome and if you're going to discipline the horse while the farrier is holding its leg up, let him know.

Shoeing horses can be a dangerous dirty job; so do not make it more difficult for the farrier. Even if the horse is well behaved when tied up and stands quietly for the farrier, stay around to be there in case you are needed. Be aware of the horse's actions and your own. Stay alert and by all means talk to the horse or chat to the farrier but don't try utilising your time by grooming the horse, the dust and the dirt has to go somewhere and it usually ends up with the farrier breathing it in. There are those horses that do not respond to kind words and feed but who still need to have their hooves attended to. Methods of restraint are available but unless you are familiar or comfortable with them do not use them, talk to the vet about sedation.

Finally a top tip regarding shoeing and equine management during the summer: Fly repellent! Nothing seems to get the horses attention more than a single fly, try not to let something so small be the cause of a dangerous situation. Horsemanship is about planning and taking pre-emptive measures. Having the horse shod should be a pleasurable part of ownership, try not to make it something for all to dread.

SHOEING

When the horse is brought in for shoeing or trimming, it should be noted how the horse is moving, whether it is lame, how the hooves are being placed upon the ground as the horse is being walked towards

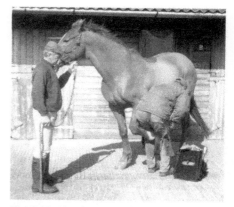

Fig. 8-13: Handlers should stand on the same side as the farrier (Photo: Alex Gill).

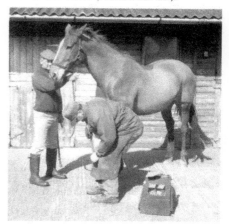

Fig. 8-14: When the farrier takes a front hoof forward, the handler should stand on the other side of the horse's head (Photo: Alex Gill).

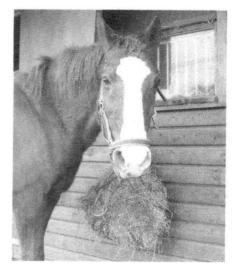

Fig. 8-15: Hay-nets can keep the horse content.

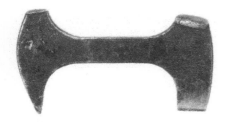

Fig. 8-16: A buffer.

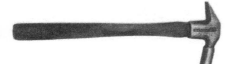

Fig. 8-17: A farriers shoeing hammer.

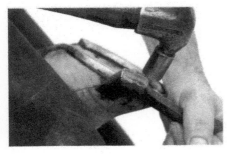

Fig. 8-18: Using the hammer and buffer to cut off the clenches, which fasten the shoes on to the hoof (Photo: J. Watts).

Fig. 8-19: A farrier's rasp.

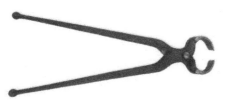

Fig. 8-20: Long handled farrier's pincers.

the observer and how the horse stands. All this can provide a lot of information and so even before the farrier has picked up a hoof, a plan of action is being formulated and decisions made by the farrier about how to approach the horse and how he will handle it.

Removing the old shoes is the first stage in shoeing; the clenches, which hold the shoe secure to the hoof must be removed. The farrier generally carries out this task using a buffer, which has a chisel shaped cutting edge (Fig. 8-16). Using the buffer in conjunction with a shoeing hammer (Fig. 8-17), the clenches are either cut off completely or raised and bent back so that as the shoe is pulled off the hoof the nails are prised out without damaging the hoof wall. To pull the shoes off without first removing the clenches makes the job more difficult, it can damage the hoof and can cause discomfort to the horse.

Removing shoes is usually one task handlers dread but there are occasions when all owners and those who care for horses need to be able to do this. Those times usually happen because a horse has partly pulled a shoe off and is likely to injure itself if it is not removed. At times like these, invariably there are some nails sticking out presenting dangerously sharp edges and as the horse may be in some discomfort it would be wise to remove these as well as any clenches still securing the shoe. This is best done by taking the hoof forwards, placing it on your knee and then rasping off any loose nails and any secure clenches. In doing that, when it comes to removing the shoe both the handler and the horse are less likely to be injured. Handlers generally have very few tools. They can probably acquire an old rasp from their farrier (Fig. 8-19) and although they may not have leather chaps or an apron to protect their legs they will definitely need to invest in a pair of long handled pincers (Fig. 8-20). These are needed to pull the shoe off and without them the job is going to be very tough.

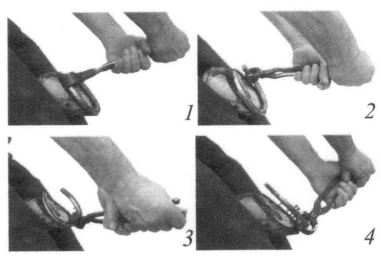

Figs. 8-21: Removing the shoe (photograph J. Watts).

When removing the shoe, using a pair of long handled pincers, start by levering at one heel, gripping the shoe and wrenching downward towards the toe of the shoe. Once the shoe has been prised away from the hoof on one side, repeat at the other heel, remembering to wrench downwards and inwards at the same time. As the shoe becomes loose, shift the positioning of the pincers and place them nearer the toe, levering towards the opposite side. Repositioning the pincers to the other side of the toe be prepared to give the shoe a final jerk and the shoe should come off (Figs. 8-21).

SHOE CHOICE

Shoes come in a wide variety of shape, size and material. Some may require fitting by a farrier more familiar with a particular type of shoe. Synthetic shoes and shoes secured by gluing techniques require skills and expertise that some farriers may not have found the need to acquire, as only a small minority of horses cannot be shod through conventional practices. The principles behind those shoes regarding hoof balance, remains the same with the exception that shoes which deform as readily as the hoof itself may prove to have benefits beyond those of steel or aluminium. This is because the shoes that can change shape instead of the hooves to which they are applied, may prove to be more beneficial for some horses with foot balance problems.

Conventional shoes, which are those formed out of metal, are available in different sizes, different weights and different designs. Even shoes that would appear to be the same to a casual observer might have subtle differences simply because a different manufacturer produces them. Despite this, most farriers choose to use a range of shoes they are familiar with and that they personally find more comfortable to use.

Nails secure metal shoes almost without exception. These are designed and shaped to assist with the precise nailing techniques required to avoid causing harm to the horse and to minimise damage to the hoof's horn. The 'square' nail has been in use by the skilled farrier for centuries and it can be driven with relative confidence. However, because in essence the nail can act as a wedge, horses going lame after shoeing are always going to be a possibility. Even when it is driven into sound horn, it is the skill of the individual farrier that makes lameness less of a probability. The nail heads are tapered and fit into a counter-sunk hole of the same shape formed within the body of the shoe. Some shoes are made out of a flat bar of metal. These are generally known as plain stamped shoes. Where the holes for the nails are stamped into a groove that is cut into the shoe, these shoes may be described as three-quarter fullered; fullering being the name of the process used to create that groove. In the UK, the majority of horses are shod using steel bar section known as fullered concave. The fullering provides grip and because the section is concave, width is achieved without the weight of the three-quarter fullered shoes. All three sections of material are used in the making of bar shoes, straight-bar shoes, egg-bar shoes and heart-bar shoes. Bar shoes are used where conventional shoes would fail to give the hoof adequate support.

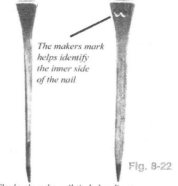

The makers mark helps identify the inner side of the nail

Fig. 8-22

The lead on the nail tip helps direct the nail to exit the hoof wall

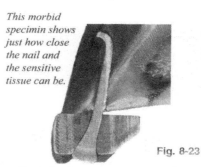

This morbid specimin shows just how close the nail and the sensitive tissue can be.

Fig. 8-23

The nail is driven through shoe and hoof.

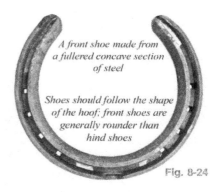

A front shoe made from a fullered concave section of steel

Shoes should follow the shape of the hoof; front shoes are generally rounder than hind shoes

Fig. 8-24

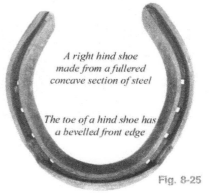

A right hind shoe made from a fullered concave section of steel

The toe of a hind shoe has a bevelled front edge

Fig. 8-25

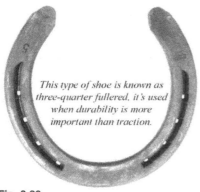

This type of shoe is known as three-quarter fullered, it's used when durability is more important than traction.

Fig. 8-26

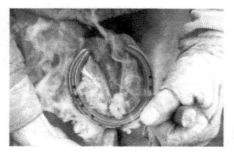

Fig. 8-29: 'Hot shoeing' is when the shoe is altered hot and the fit of the shoe is checked against the hoof, while the shoe is still warm.

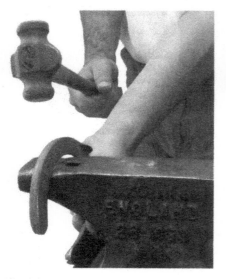

Fig. 8-30: 'Cold shoeing' is when the shoes are fitted without the use of heat to make the shoes more pliable. Most metal shoes can be altered cold (Photo: J. Watts).

Straight-bar shoes are seldom in use but egg-bar shoes are used to support the hoof at the heels and so are commonly seen on horses with collapsed heel or navicular problems. Heart-bar shoes are also used on horses with flat feet and low heels but are also associated with laminitis; in essence, they are used where the frog is used to take load away from the hoof wall.

SHOE FITTING

When fitting both bar shoes and conventional shoes the same principles are applied. All shoes require that they are fitted so that they permit the foot to follow the direction of the flight pattern of motion directed by the geometric structure of the limb. To place a symmetrical shoe upon an asymmetric foot would make as much sense as wearing our left shoes on our right feet. Adequate width and length to the shoes fitted is an absolute essential. Thought has to be given about how those feet will change shape in the coming days and weeks. Fitting the shoes 'tight' or 'close' will not accommodate for new growth which will push the shoe forwards and as it does so, short shoes or tight fitting shoes will no longer do their job but instead are likely to cause damage.

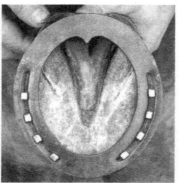

Fig. 8-27: The 'egg-bar' shoe extends further back than an open heeled shoe.

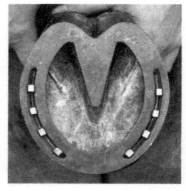

Fig. 8-28: The 'heart bar' shoe uses a triangular shaped plate to reduce the weight applied to the hoof wall.

Bar shoes are fitted in the same way although they are much harder to fit and this is because effectively they are a complete circle, therefore as they are altered on one aspect of the shoe they also alter on another. This means they do require a greater skill if they are to be fitted accurately. This added skill coupled with the skills and time required to make them or the extra cost of buying them transforms the cost to the owner to double that which they would pay for conventional shoeing.

There are two principal methods of fitting the shoes and they are defined as 'hot shoeing' and 'cold shoeing'. Hot shoeing is where the shoe is placed upon the hoof to check its fit and then altered while the shoe is still hot. During fitting, the shoe is often burnt on to the hoof and this is thought by some to provide a better fit than cold shoeing.

136

However, the time involved in fitting is, of necessity, more hurried because the farrier must work at speed while the heat remains in the shoe. In cold shoeing as the shoes are altered cold some sections of steel can prove difficult to alter but with those sections of steel which can be altered cold, it can be argued that more time and care can be taken to achieve an exact fit. Both practices have their pros and cons but the reality is that both methods are only as good as the farrier doing the job.

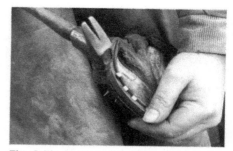

Fig. 8-31: As the nail is driven through the shoe and hoof, the point of the nail should exit the wall.

NAILING ON

At the start of fixing the shoe on, the farrier will hold the first nail in position with one hand at the same time directing it in to the horny hoof and with the other hand, drive it in with a hammer. It is because the nails are driven into the hoof at an angle that the shoe has a tendency to drift away from the desired location. This can be something of a problem when using shoes without clips, but with shoes that have clips forged into them or welded on to the shoe, this is less problematic. When nailing on shoes without clips the first nail to be placed into the hoof will be at the heel. In that position, the nail is driven in at less of an angle and the shoe drifts less. With shoes with clips, a nail closer to the toe is the first to be hammered into position. There the hoof is set at a more acute angle so the drift would be more without the clips holding the shoe in place. As each nail is driven into the hoof, the nail is aimed to emerge out of the hoof at a point somewhere between 1.5cm – 2.5cm from the ground surface of the foot. Each nail is tipped with a lead, which encourages the nail to exit the hoof at the desired height. Damaged nails or rusty nails are not recommended for use as these do not behave in a given way and so can result in the nail being liable to exit too soon or interfere with sensitive tissue. The amount of nail exiting the hoof will vary according to what size nail is used but whatever the amount; it needs to be made safe. Horses are strong and often unpredictable and as the farrier has to hold the foot while he works on the hoof, exposed nail points are liable to cause injury to the farrier so these points are quickly removed or made safe. This task is generally done by using the claw of the shoeing hammer. The nail is slotted between the claws and twisted off.

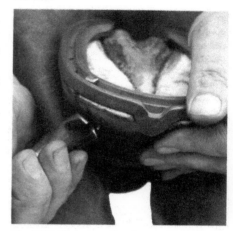

Fig. 8-32: To remove the sharp nail points and make task more safe, the tips are twisted off.

FINISHING OFF

When the nails have been driven securely into the shoe and hoof, the foot is taken forwards and placed on the farrier's knee or on the shoeing stand. In that position the cut nails protruding from the hoof wall are neatly rasped to give them a short uniform length. Horn is then removed from under the nail segments, forming a cut recess in the hoof wall and the nails are then folded down into the recess to form a 'clench'. The clench is the portion of the nails that keeps the shoe

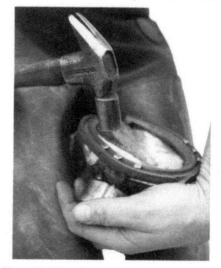

Fig. 8-33: When the final nail is in place and it's point twisted off, the nails are driven in tightly. At the same time the cropped end of the nail is bent away from the hoof wall; this will form the clench (Photo: J. Watts).

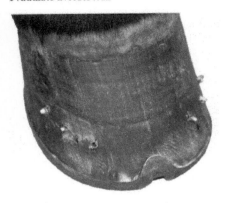

Fig. 8-34: Here the nails have been driven through the shoe and the hoof, and the nail points removed. The small portion of nail that protudes from the hoof wall will be made even and bent over to form the clench (Photo: J. Watts).

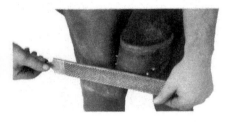

Fig. 8-35: The cut nails are rasped to an even length, then a notch of horn is removed directly below. This recess will allow the finished clench to lie flush with the hoof wall (Photo: J. Watts).

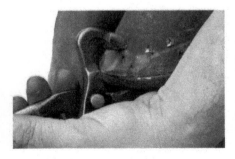

Fig. 8-36: When the recess has been cut into the hoof wall, the clenches are formed by pulling, or hammering the short square shaped segments of nail so that they claps the shoe firmly to the hoof. When that procedure is complete, they can be rasped smooth (Photo: J. Watts).

securely fastened to the hoof. Once the clenches have been formed, they and any other features affecting the overall appearance of the finished work are rasped smooth. On the hind feet where often two clips are forged into the shoe and the toe of the shoe is set back on the hoof, the toe section of the hoof is allowed to protrude beyond the edge of the shoe and is neatly rounded off. Hind shoes are often set back as a safety feature should the horse overreach; this is to try to ensure any damage to the bulbs of the heel on the forefoot is as minimal as possible.

LAME HORSES

It would seem inevitable that occasionally some horses can go lame after shoeing. This is generally because some aspect of the sole could be touching the shoe, or a nail either has penetrated sensitive tissue or has been positioned so close as to inflict pain. If this occurs, the matter should be discussed with the farrier who has shod the horse. If the lameness did not become apparent until after the farrier had left the yard he should be contacted immediately and his advice sought.

If sensitive tissue has been damaged (nail prick) it is likely that it would be identified instantly. This type of injury is uncommon and when it does occur, it does not normally present a serious lasting problem. Nail binds are due to the nailing positioned close to the sensitive tissue. This type of injury may not become apparent for some hours by which time the farrier could be tens of miles away and not contactable, or the horse could be turned out in a field with any lameness simply not being detected. A similar scenario is applicable if the sole is in contact with the shoe. The farrier would spot obvious cases while he was still working on the horse but again, sometimes it may be a few hours before the horse becomes noticeably unsound. All these types of injuries occur because of understandable human errors of judgement, although if it happens too frequently with any one particular farrier then obviously the standard of his or her work has to be questioned. However, it is the combined complexity of the hoof and the almost naive crudeness of driving nails in to what is effectively a thick piece of skin, which means that the chances of something going wrong are ever present. Of course the other added variable that increases the probability of lameness after shoeing is also one of the primary reasons hooves need attention and that is that they change shape under the weight of the horse they are supporting. This is why the horse can be sound when the farrier leaves the yard but lame some hours later. Therefore, as lameness is an ever-present scenario after shoeing, it would be advantageous for all owners and handlers (as highlighted earlier in this chapter) to be able to remove shoes themselves because the farrier may not always be there.

Identifying lameness is a skill, which is acquired through experience. Farriers are not specifically trained to identify and diagnose lameness whereas veterinarians are. However, usually the owners and handlers are the first to spot any problems. This is because not only are they are likely to be the first on site but also because they are the ones who often know their horse better than anyone else and so are more 'in tune' with their animal's normal behaviour. All horses, like people, seem to have their own pain threshold levels, which can affect the time-scale of some lameness' becoming apparent. The first and general sign is the loss of fluid symmetry of movement within the usage of the limbs and unequal weight bearing. As the animal stands, it may be noticed that he will adopt a 'pointing' stance that is, resting a foreleg in advance of the sound limb, that foreleg being placed vertically beneath the animal's centre of mass and supporting the majority of the horse's weight. In long-term lamenesses, the hoof of the sound limb can become noticeably larger. Resting a hind limb is normal but if the animal chooses to rest one hind limb for long periods then that is not normal. An acutely lame horse will hold his hoof off the ground and show a strong reluctance to bear any weight on it at all; these animals are clearly easier to identify than others are. It is the asymmetry of movement, which is the strong diagnostic agent, used to define which limb and for the trained observer, even the site and possible cause, may be identified. Trotting a horse both toward and away from an observer allows that person to see just how the animal is moving. This is better carried out on a hard even surface. The trot in theory is a symmetrical gait and so therefore is used as a diagnostic gait of choice. The trot produces the speed, spring and concussive forces that usually reveal the lameness. The horse needs to be trotted by a handler in a straight line, over a longer distance rather than a short one. The horse needs to be allowed to move freely with the handler applying little or no force through the lead rope giving the animal's head an unrestrained range of motion as holding the lead rope taut can also cause the animal to move crookedly. Head motion is very diagnostic. If the horse is lame in front, as the painful limb bears weight as the hoof contacts the ground, his head and neck will rise. Watching the head raise the instant the hoof contacts the ground can be quite a difficult task as it is about linking the footfall to head motion. Hind limb lameness is more difficult to identify. In these cases, the head will tend to go down as the hoof of the lame limb contacts the ground. This is done in an effort to shift the animal's bodyweight forwards transferring weight off the affected limb. Hip motion is also diagnostic but difficult to see. Here the hip may rise as the affected limb is asked to bear weight. There is in fact a whole range of techniques, which can used to identify, which limb is affected. Although for the farrier or handler on their own, simply turning the horse in tight circles first one way and then the other should display a pattern of movement that will identify quite readily acute-type lamenesses associated with post shoeing.

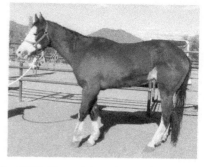

Fig. 8-37: The pointing stance; this is where the horse rests a forelimb by placing it in advance of the sound, weight-bearing, foreleg. (Photo, courtesy Arizona Equine Rescue Organization).

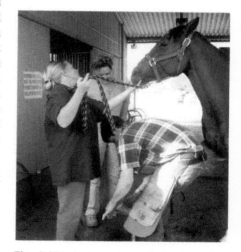

Fig. 8-38: Hoofcare is, and should be the result of, an uninhibited cooperation and understanding between owner, farrier and vet.

Here the three parties are seen working together; their objective to provide the best care they knowingly can give. (Photo, courtesy Arizona Equine Rescue Organization).

FARRIER, VET AND CLIENT RELATIONS

It is generally when horses become lame that owner, farrier and veterinary relationships are put to the test, as each have very different roles. Each need to remember that farriery is not the sole domain of the farrier and neither is it the farrier's sole responsibility. It is the owners who play the most active role in farriery, as it is they who decide when, where and by whom their horses are to be shod. So if you're an owner, the responsibility for the management of the horse is yours and it is you who will constantly need to consider that their daily management routines will affect both the hoof shape and determine the frequency of trimming and shoeing.

Here in the UK, farrier and vet relationships have had a long and at times uneasy history. Undoubtedly, much of this has been due to social, educational and economic divides. However, the same could be said about the farrier / owner affiliation. Communication is the key along with mutual respect and acknowledgement. Better farriery education and new technology will also help to define the boundaries between the two roles of farrier and vet. For centuries farriery has been a craft and an art but not a science. When it becomes a science, developed through a systematic study that defines observable material facts, then farriers will establish a new image and a new role. It is because of its workman-like image and the fact that the vast majority of accepted trials and studies into farriery have been carried out by the veterinary colleges that the two roles have become confused. In the USA, the approach to tackle the problem of farrier / vet relations has been to combine teaching and research facilities and it would be hoped this approach would be adopted worldwide. However, practically all problems within the farriery industry could be removed if issues regarding motivation, training, continuing education and remuneration were all addressed. Many of those issues seem destined to haunt the industry ad infinitum. Hopefully however, those who read this book will understand the need we all have to acquire the wider knowledge necessary to help overcome many of the obstacles that prevent us all from acting in unison to ensure that horses receive the best farriery attention. There is an analogy to be made here regarding the constraints of a free market. Take a look at the car tyre industry. Tyres are made and can be fitted to your cars that provide better, safer traction whatever the terrain. Certain tyres can reduce aquaplaning, others can reduce road noise and some, when correctly fitted and balanced, can increase the life of your car, but whenever we need new tyres, we phone round to get the cheapest! Unfortunately, the same parallels are to be found in farriery today. However, in farriery the lowest charge does not necessarily mean poorest work and the most expensive fee does not always guarantee a first-class job. The only certainty is that poor workmanship is too high a price to pay and will always prove the most expensive and it is those who pay the bills who will shape this industry's future.

OUR PACT WITH THE HORSE

Riding gives great pleasure but it must be accepted that owning and caring for a horse is also a great responsibility and something not to be taken lightly. The horse needs a great deal of knowledgeable care and attention and the more it is ridden the more it is liable to need expert care and this includes shoeing.

The horse is one of the few creatures in this world which is universally valued, loved and admired. It is an animal that has helped shape landscapes, build civilisations, forge nations and defend empires. Cultures have evolved, exist and owe their survival to the horse. Here in the UK and other English speaking nations lives and industries revolve around its being. Its beauty and majesty has inspired artists for thousands upon thousands of years, from cave artists to artist/anatomists like Da Vinci and Stubbs. So we who are passionate about it have a duty and an obligation to do our best by the horse whatever our role: long may it remain with us and as custodians long may we serve.

THE AUTHOR'S FINAL WORD

I could tell you all about the horse, what shape its hooves should be, how each joint in its complex anatomy performs but still you would not know the essentials of farriery.

To understand what farriery is and what it is not and to realise the truth behind all the actions you must experience its practices. I hope this book helps you with your journey and makes your involvement with the horse a more, rewarding, fulfilling and satisfying experience.

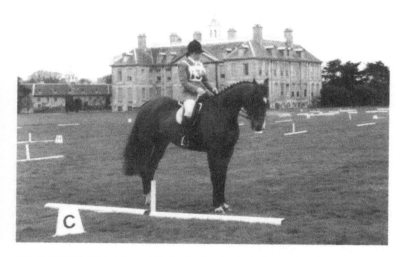

Fig. 8-38: Sally Chiarella and Doric; the inspiration behind this book. (Photo, J. Motley).

Bibliography

'If you take ideas from one source it's called plagiarism. When you take ideas from five its called research'

Craig, M., *Hoof Adaptability* (EponaShoe Inc.) http://www.eponashoe.com/Documents/HoofAdaptability.htm (Access March 2007)

Danvers, C., *Horse Holding 101* http://www.foxtailforge.com/infosheethorseholding.shtml (Access March 2007)

Parks, A., *In-depth: Palmar Foot Pain: Structure and Function of the Equine Digit in Relation to Palmar Foot Pain* (AAEP Proceedings / Vol. 52 / 2006, p188-187)

Savoldi, M.T., Rosenberg, G.F., *Uniform Sole Thickness* http://farrierart.com/Uniform%20Sole%20Thickness%20-%20Michael%20Savoldi%203%20pages.pdf (Access March 2007)

van Heel, M.C.V., *Distal limb development and effects of shoeing techniques on limb dynamics of today's equine athlete* (© M.C.V. van Heel, 2005)

Index